THE
NO-HYSTERECTOMY
OPTION

THE NO-HYSTERECTOMY OPTION

Your Body—Your Choice

Revised and Updated

Herbert A. Goldfarb, M.D.
with Judith Greif, R.N., F.N.P., C., M.S.

John Wiley & Sons, Inc.

New York · Chichester · Weinheim · Brisbane · Singapore · Toronto

Published by John Wiley & Sons, Inc.

Library of Congress Cataloging-in-Publication Data

Goldfarb, Herbert A.
    The no-hysterectomy option : your body—your choice / Herbert A.
Goldfarb, with Judith Greif. — Rev. and updated.
        p.   cm.
    Previously published: 1990.
    Includes bibliographical references and index.
    ISBN 0-471-16557-3 (paper : alkpaper)
    1. Hysterectomy—Popular works. 2. Hysterectomy—Decision making.
I. Greif, Judith. II. Title.
RG391.G64   1997
618.1'453—dc21   96–29848
                                                                  CIP

Printed in the United States of America
10 9 8 7 6 5 4 3 2 1

To our families . . .

To Laurence, who inspired this book and continues to teach by example.

To Leslie, who gives more love per square inch than any person I know.

To Robert Drew, who already has made us proud.

To Lisa, whose dreams are becoming reality and who continues to soar.

To Steve, who provides love, stability, and energy for the dream.

To Scott, whose success makes me smile and whose potential makes me bullish.

To Beverly, my love, who provides the rudder for our ship and the beacon of our purpose.

For my mother and father, who inspired me to go as far as I could. Quitting and failure were never part of their vocabulary. Success meant being satisfied that you've done your very best.

To Judith Greif, who began as a co-writer and became a very close friend. Thank you.

H.G.

* * *

To Ruth, my sister and best friend, whom I respect tremendously for her courage, and whose success, wit, and wisdom I strive to emulate. Without you, this book would never have been a reality.

To my mother and father, in gratitude for the selfless generosity, patience, encouragement, guidance, love, and support that only nurturing parents can provide.

To Samantha, age seven, who was born a month after the first version of this book was born. You continue to be a never-ending source of pride and joy.

And to Joe, my Don Quixote, who showed me that dreams are not impossible and that windmills fuel a love that is boundless.

J.G.

CONTENTS

8 WHEN HYSTERECTOMY IS UNAVOIDABLE 137

PART THREE

THE AFTERMATH—
TAKING BACK CONTROL
OF YOUR BODY

9 COPING WITH THE AFTERMATH 159

PREFACE

As to diseases, make a habit of two things: to help or at least not to harm.

—HIPPOCRATES, 400 B.C.

Before I was born, I had a sister whom I will never know, because in the days before the routine use of antibiotics, she died of sepsis following a so-called routine tonsillectomy. My late mother went on to have two sons, and while she certainly loved us, she frequently lamented the loss of her only daughter. Her daughter was taken from her unnecessarily at a time when tonsillectomy was common. We now know the importance of tonsils to the immune system, and the dangers of unwarranted operations. Perhaps my sister's death was not entirely in vain, because through my deeply personal and tragic experience, I have become particularly sensitized to a cavalier approach to surgery. Hundreds of thousands of women are told each year that a hysterectomy is necessary. Perhaps you or a loved one will be among those people who have been or will be offered hysterectomy as a panacea for your gynecological problems. It is for you that I am writing this book. While we do not have all of the answers yet, I hope I will stimulate you to ask the right questions and help you to make the best, most informed decision for yourself. It is my fervent hope that this book will help women to avoid unnecessary hysterectomy, but there is more to it than that.

When I first undertook this project, the main thrust of this book was telling women how and why to avoid hysterectomies. However, as I became more involved in its research and writing, I realized that there is much more to say. As a result, this book took on a much broader perspective, although its central focus remains hysterectomy. It is now a book about the physical and psychological aspects of women's health. It is an attempt to thoroughly discuss all of the principal conditions that can and have resulted in major abdominal surgery for women. It discusses in detail what these conditions are, how they have been diagnosed and treated in the past, and what new and future therapies are becoming available. The new therapies I have recommended consider the total woman, not merely her pelvic organs. My aim is to help equip you with maximal knowledge and understanding of a serious medical problem so that you can make a truly informed decision regarding its management. It is my strong conviction that you should be a partner in your care with your physician and not just a passive recipient.

Years ago, when a pregnant woman went into labor, she was placed flat on her back and given a pharmacopoeia of painkillers and "twilight sleep" preparations to sedate her until it was finally time to whisk her off to the delivery room. There, she'd be strapped down, placed under general anesthesia, and her baby delivered while an anxious father paced the hall-ways. The baby would be routinely injected with Narcan to reverse its nar-cotic stupor and moved into the nursery. Later, the mother could "visit" her baby, but only during specified hours. Today, women walk until active labor begins. If they wish, mothers are fully alert and unmedicated throughout the birth of their children, which often takes place in homelike birthing rooms. Fathers are encouraged to participate in their wives' labor and to be present during the delivery. In effect, women no longer unquestioningly accept or even tolerate the passive role to which they were delegated during child-birth a generation ago. As a result, obstetrical philosophy and practice has changed dramatically. Now it is time for gynecology to follow suit.

Hysterectomy is the second most frequently performed major opera-tion in the United States—even though half the population (men) never re-quire this surgery. According to recent statistics, more than 35 percent of women over the age of fifty have had a hysterectomy. And, tragically, 65 percent of the time, the surgery is performed between ages thirty and fifty, a time when many of these women are still in their reproductive years. Add to that the horrifying fact that over two thousand women die from hys-terectomies annually, and another 240,000 suffer major complications. The numbers become especially staggering in light of the evidence uncovered by numerous analyses of these procedures: From 90 to 95 percent of these surgeries are elective!

In their 1979 book, *Understanding Hysterectomy: A Woman's Guide,* Drs. Giustini and Keefer wrote:

> Most people have known someone who continues to bleed from the uterus no matter what the doctor tries. Flooding causing so-cial embarrassment, or the necessity of wearing a pad two or more weeks monthly, are problems for which women want solu-tions. Most doctors try hormone therapy or repeated D&Cs (scraping of the womb) to correct or control these troublesome complaints. After a woman has had three or more D&Cs, or has taken several courses of hormone therapy, the patient tires of the "conservative" approach. She wants something done. Hysterec-tomy is definitive, corrective, and permanent treatment. Often no abnormal tissue is found in the removal of the uterus, but clearly that did not mean the operation was unnecessary.

The opinions expressed by Giustini and Keefer in many ways reflect a mentality that pervaded the medical community less than twenty years ago.

In fairness, options were limited in 1979. Unfortunately, however, this mind-set is still with us today—that a hysterectomy is a relatively risk-free panacea for the woman who is troubled by a gynecologic problem, has completed her family, and wants to eliminate the nuisance of menstruation. Nothing could be farther from the truth.

All major surgery is fraught with complications. Hysterectomy is no exception, sometimes resulting in hemorrhage, urinary tract trauma, intestinal injuries, posthysterectomy depression, sexual dysfunction, early ovarian failure, heart disease, and osteoporosis. Writing in a 1994 issue of *Obstetrics and Gynecology Clinics of North America* concerning the indications for hysterectomy, Drs. Ravnikar and Chen alerted fellow physicians to the staggering and sobering facts that the complication rates for traditional types of hysterectomies ranged from 24 percent for vaginal to 43 percent for abdominal procedures. They went on to caution that even the newer type of laparoscopic-assisted vaginal hysterectomy (LAVH) resulted in complications because physicians needed to learn how to properly perform this difficult operation. Performed correctly, no complications should arise; however, even the finest, most skilled surgeon needs careful training before attempting laparoscopic surgery.

This book is about changing the idea that hysterectomy is the "definitive therapy" for women's pelvic complaints—and it's about discovering options. It reexamines the propriety of hysterectomy and questions traditional medical practice. It challenges when hysterectomy is "indicated" versus when it is truly necessary, primarily from the woman's perspective, to safeguard her life or substantially improve its quality.

I remember back in the 1960s when my mother-in-law announced that she had just come from visiting her gynecologist. He had told her that "it was time she had a hysterectomy." He had said that her problems were minor, but that after a woman reaches age 40, she really "ought to" have a hysterectomy because "it would save a lot of trouble later on." Fortunately, her son-in-law advised her to the contrary.

We need to revise our thinking that hysterectomy is benign and convenient, and that there is no other hope for women faced with certain gynecologic problems. As we will see, hysterectomy is far from benign, and there is certainly a great deal of hope and reason for optimism about maintaining a woman's reproductive ability.

Unlike the medical practitioners of the past, we know that the uterus is more than a receptacle for the fetus. While we still do not completely comprehend the role of the uterus, our lack of understanding is not a valid reason for removing it. Yet hysterectomies are performed well over a half million times each year in North America. The cost of hysterectomy is too high—physically, emotionally, sexually, and economically—for anyone to accept it without considering the many options to having one's uterus removed.

It is true that many women express no untoward aftereffects as a result of hysterectomy, but others reveal significant depression over the removal of their uterus. The medical literature is replete with reports not only of physical complications but of emotional problems developing after hysterectomy. Fortunately, we now possess a much better understanding of what happens to women when they have a hysterectomy, and we have much improved modalities for coping with the devastation that often follows.

I came to realize that we had to calculate a risk/reward ratio to identify which patients would suffer from the performance of the procedure. The more I thought about this, the more I reasoned that one of the most important things that I could do was to help women stay healthy and avoid frivolous hysterectomy at all cost.

Beginning in the early 1970s, several new technologies were developed and/or perfected that have made a big difference in uterine preservation. For example, the hysteroscope (a fiberoptic tube that is inserted into the uterus through the cervix without the need to make an incision; see Chapter 3) allowed doctors to view the inside of a uterus to diagnose and treat certain abnormal conditions without the need for more invasive surgery. The laser offered treatment for abnormal uterine bleeding that was preferable to hysterectomy.

In the seven years since the first edition of this book was published, changes in gynecologic practice have been overwhelming. While laser treatment was the up-and-coming technique in 1990, its use today has fallen out of favor. There has been a rediscovery of basic surgical instruments, such as very sharp, disposable scissors, which are less expensive than the laser and more comfortable for surgeons to use because they fall into place with original surgical training. Other new techniques have allowed us to present significant alternatives to our patients. These include new hormonal therapies such as the GnRH agonist, which controls vaginal hemorrhage and reduces the size of uterine tumors. Myomectomy certainly offers an extremely palatable alternative to hysterectomy, and in combination with the use of the new GnRH agonist, we can reduce the size of myomas (fibroids) to the point where they can be easily removed with minimal blood loss. Laparoscopic myomectomy is now a reality because of advanced suturing and tissue removal systems. Utilizing these techniques, along with the advancements we have made in laparoscopic surgery or just careful observation, may allow us to eliminate as many as one-half to two-thirds of the hysterectomies performed each year!

After the first edition of this book was published in 1990, I traveled around the country speaking to women's groups. I was deluged by women with horror stories about how their lives were radically changed by hysterectomy. These women voiced two predominant and recurring points: First, hysterectomy was a negative event in their lives—the adverse effects of which could not easily be reversed. Second, they had been told repeatedly, "And while we're in there, we will also remove your ovaries." This was usually done to minimize the risk of ovarian cancer. (Contrary to what you might think, it does not eliminate the risk entirely, because cancer cells can still be present after the ovaries are removed.) And unfortunately, many women taking estrogen replacement therapy after oophorectomy (removal of the ovaries) still suffered with physical as well as psychological symptoms. The controversy concerning ovarian cancer has not gone away, but I strongly believe that it has been overstated. The unhappiness after oophorectomy still outweighs the potential risk of ovarian cancer. This is especially true now that we can use endovaginal ultrasound to monitor patients at risk (see Chapter 8).

Meeting these women and hearing their stories gave me the impetus to continue to search for new techniques to offer patients. I wanted to offer a fresh approach to women who wanted to preserve their reproductive organs, but who were often intimidated into undergoing hysterectomy.

In 1990 I attended an advanced endoscopic conference in Switzerland where a single event changed my life: A French physician showed a brief film of a new procedure during which he inserted the tip of a laser fiber into a fibroid to destroy it. This five-minute video helped to change my outlook and approach to fibroid management dramatically. I sat transfixed because I felt that I was witnessing an extraordinary and potentially revolutionary new treatment. On my return home, I conducted the first U.S. procedures and coined the term "myoma coagulation" or "myolysis" (see Chapter 3). Over the last six years I have performed hundreds of these procedures and have published in the medical literature. I have lectured and taught this technique to physicians throughout the United States. The evolution in gynecologic surgery from laser to electrocautery has made this and other procedures more user-friendly. Still, there are many doubters. New ideas travel slowly in the medical community. I am pleased and proud to say that I have personally saved hundreds of women from hysterectomies.

This book goes beyond helping women to understand more about their bodies and to demand more of their physicians for the sake of avoiding major surgery. It is also about minimizing the impact of a chronic condition on a woman's lifestyle so that she can avoid major upheavals in her career and personal life.

During the Victorian era, the weak and wan female was a popular image. Perhaps because they posed a threat to their male contemporaries, intelligent and active women might be told that they suffered from hysteria or so-called neurasthenia and that they must take a "rest cure." This involved taking to her bed for weeks or even months, during which time the woman couldn't read, write, or enjoy any social contact. That this alleged "cure" itself could actually induce madness is documented in one account by a noted feminist of the time, Charlotte Perkins Gilman, who wrote a famous story about her experience called *The Yellow Wallpaper*.

Women no longer desire or tolerate prolonged idle periods of recuperation. In addition, they expect to play an active role in maintaining or restoring their health. They want to be out of the hospital quickly and back on their feet so that they can resume work and family life. To help you meet these goals, this book shows you a myriad of new medical and surgical techniques in gynecologic care for urinary incontinence, uterine prolapse, endometriosis, menopausal symptoms, osteoporosis, abnormal bleeding from fibroids, and other conditions. It offers advice on how nutrition, exercise, and psychotherapy can help you to keep mind and body sound whether you are attempting to avoid hysterectomy or cope with its aftermath. I hope that it will help you to make the best, most informed decisions about your health.

ACKNOWLEDGMENTS

A great many people, including friends, family members, and colleagues, were indispensable in supporting us through this undertaking. They served as resources and sounding boards, as well as offered time, advice, encouragement, and moral support. To them we are greatly indebted.

This book involved a tremendous amount of research. We especially thank the staff of the Health Sciences Library of the Tishman Learning Center, Montefiore Medical Center, Bronx, New York, for assisting in this task. In particular, Josie Lim, Deborah Green, and Vernon Bruette were unwavering sources of assistance and information. In addition, we thank Ann Marie Palladino for facilitating a computer search of the literature that saved hours of tedious manual work.

For assistance in preparing the manuscript, including proofreading, editing, and photocopying, we acknowledge Joseph Pedreiro, a seasoned professional in these and other tasks.

We extend our gratitude to Rachel Feldblum for her helpful professional guidance in the section concerning emotional issues related to hysterectomy.

Finally, we commend and acknowledge the staff at John Wiley & Sons, especially David Sobel, Ruth Greif, Ted Scheffler, Judith McCarthy, and Joanne Palmer, for their invaluable assistance in making this book the best it could be.

Special Acknowledgments

I wish to acknowledge the influences on my life that gave me the courage to keep going and "get it done":

- My teachers at New York University College of Medicine, who taught me not to compromise excellence.
- Saul Farber, M.D., who never let me forget that humanism in medicine accompanies excellence.
- Sophie Kleegman, M.D. I was one of those who listened.
- Charles Debrovner, M.D., whose friendship has been cherished, and whose honesty, strength of character, and achievement have been an inspiration.
- Milton Goldrath, M.D., who had patience and time for me and helped change my life.

- Franklin Loffer, M.D., whose kindness and excellence were a source of unbelievable help.
- Douglas Phillips, M.D., whose counsel is invaluable and whose friendship is treasured.
- Anthony Oropollo, M.D., for continuing his staunch support when I need him most.
- Marie Oropollo, who is always there for me. I'll never forget your help.
- Emily Murphy, for being there with an open door and an open ear and having the courage to see the light.
- Judith Greif, R.N.C., whose friendship is among the most important byproducts of this book.
- Stanley Goldfarb, M.D., who has set an example of excellence and showed me that it could be done.
- My mother, whose persistence and strength of character gave me the will to go on. Her love and support never wavered.
- My father, whose life was a textbook of determination and character. I wish you were here to share this with me.
- To my wife, Beverly Susan, who can never be thanked enough for being there to share the good times and support me through the hard ones.

Herbert A. Goldfarb, M.D.

THE
NO-HYSTERECTOMY
OPTION

PART ONE

THE HYSTERECTOMY CONTROVERSY

By eight o'clock we were in the operating room. Once in the OR, how did I feel? I felt important. . . . There is something about a uniform, too, that makes one feel important. My whole being reeked of my station. I was an insider. I looked just like the others. I had a place, a job, and I was being taught the secrets of medicine. If we had expressed our feelings of elitism, we might have said, "How terrible never to see the inside of the OR, never to have a role in the drama there." I was ashamed of the power I felt in that room, ashamed of what I was becoming, and yet I was also enjoying it.
    —MICHELLE HARRISON, M.D., *A Woman in Residence*

1

DO YOU REALLY NEED
A HYSTERECTOMY?

*My experience has been that if your condition is not life-
threatening, most doctors don't take it very seriously. Friends
and clients have echoed my sentiments. When will the esteemed
physicians learn that the quality of a person's life is as
important as its length?*
> —SUSAN LIPPMAN, "Lament for a Lost Uterus"

You are probably reading this book because you (or someone you care about) have been told that you "need" a hysterectomy. Every year in this country, doctors perform tens of thousands of avoidable hysterectomies. You may be able to preserve your precious pelvic organs if you know about the many new alternatives to hysterectomy that are now available, and if you know how to find a doctor who will respect your wishes and who is skilled at providing these options to you. Most of this book is devoted to understanding the conditions that sometimes lead women to hysterectomy and the possible ways to avoid the surgery, but it is both interesting and important to understand the history behind the evolution of women's surgery—in other words, how all these unnecessary hysterectomies came to be done in the first place.

THE HISTORICAL PERSPECTIVE

In *Dr. W. A. Evans' How to Keep Well Book*, published in the United States in 1917, the author explains the cure for syphilis, which he said may be contracted through the use of an "unclean towel" or "toilet." He recommended "one injection of neosalvarsan . . . followed by six months of mercury injections . . . three more injections of neosalvarsan . . . followed by [two additional years of] mercury injected twice each week . . . [and] mercury by mouth." We now know, of course, that antibiotics—usually peni-

3

cillin—are the only effective treatment for syphilis. Worse still, we know that excess intake of mercury can lead to insanity (Mad Hatter's Disease) and even to death. Here, then, is one case where the cure was as bad as if not worse than the disease.

Obviously, medicine is an ever-evolving science, where practices and opinions about what may be "necessary and indicated" for a particular disease process change with the times. This chapter will give you a brief overview of the medical perspective on women's health and the evolution of women's surgery, and it will discuss how this has led to the trends and controversies we see today concerning hysterectomy.

According to the 1994 National Hospital Discharge Survey (an annual probability sampling of hospital discharges of patients admitted to nonfederal, short-stay hospitals within the United States) (Wilcox, 1994), hysterectomy remains the most common non-pregnancy-related surgery performed on women. It outdistances tonsillectomy, cholecystectomy (removal of the gallbladder), hernia repair, and even coronary bypass surgery. It is also one of the most ancient of surgeries. The Greek physician Archigenes was said to have performed hysterectomy in Rome in the first century A.D. And ironically enough, unlike most other things in Western medicine (such as the treatment of syphilis mentioned before), hysterectomy has remained relatively unchanged throughout nearly two millennia.

The first obstetrician-gynecologists were women: the priestesses and healers of ancient Sumer, Assyria, Egypt, and Greece who attended births. Throughout the Middle Ages, through the Renaissance, and up to the Industrial Age, obstetrics, through the practice of midwifery, remained the exclusive domain of the female practitioner. Medicine, as learned in universities by male physicians during the Middle Ages, was intimately tied to religion. The practice of midwifery, however, began to be perceived by society as founded in superstition. Rather than being tied to religion, it began to be associated with witchcraft, which was viewed as evil and demonic.

These notions paved the way for male physicians to become involved for the first time in obstetrics, and by association in gynecology. However, this practice was not condoned by many in the medical field. In her book, *Men Who Control Women's Health*, Diane Scully quotes Dr. Samuel Gregory as writing, around 1848, to implore physicians to abandon midwifery because:

> the introduction of men into the lying-in chamber, in place of female attendants, has increased the suffering and dangers of childbearing women, and brought multiplied injuries and fatalities upon mothers and children; it violates the sensitive feelings of husbands and wives, and causes an untold amount of domes-

tic misery; the unlimited intimacy between a numerous profession and the female population silently and effectually wears away female delicacy and professional morality, and tends, probably more than any other cause in existence, to undermine the foundation of public virtue.

Sadly, medical and social practices of the mid-1800s made this true. Early nineteenth-century physicians lacked knowledge of anesthesia and antibiotics, worked with primitive instruments, and until Dr. Ignaz Semmelweis linked the often-fatal childbed fever to inadequate hygiene on the part of physicians, often went from the autopsy room to the bedchamber without washing their equipment or their hands. As a result, physicians themselves—unlike midwives, who were not involved in dissecting corpses—often spread death and disease from household to household by serving as the vehicles through which bacteria were transmitted. At the same time, Victorian morals precluded complete and proper examinations of female genitalia. During the 1800s, it was considered inappropriate and unscrupulous for male physicians to examine women, except by reaching up under the women's skirts while averting their eyes! This practice continued in some circles even after the invention of the speculum. In 1848 Dr. Charles Meigs wrote, "I am proud to say . . . that there are women who prefer to suffer the extremity of danger and pain rather than waive those scruples of delicacy which prevent their maladies from being fully explored."

Before the nineteenth century, female sexuality was never acknowledged to be important, unique, or worthy of study. In the 1800s, for the first time in modern Western history, female sexuality was not only the focus of male interest, and even of men's fear and loathing, but it became as well a force that could be controlled surgically. As a result, women then ran the risk of having their lives placed in jeopardy by operative practices stemming from the need of male physicians to intervene. It was during this time that hysterectomy and oophorectomy (removal of the ovaries) came into vogue as the cure for nearly everything ailing women, including headaches, epilepsy, indigestion, backache, liver trouble, and, of course, "excessive sexual desire."

Then, as now, there was controversy and conflicting opinions among male doctors regarding the preservation of the uterus. Some physicians viewed the female in the almost revered role of childbearer. One doctor even went so far as to say that "the Almighty, in creating the female sex, had taken a uterus and built up a woman around it." In 1873 Dr. Edward H. Clarke, a physician and Harvard professor, cautioned against a college education for women because it would cause "uterine atrophy." Women were socialized to be docile, feeble, and subservient to men. If they were not, then medicine had to intervene; and despite their importance to the sanctity of childbearing, the female organs must be sacrificed.

From Hippocrates who said "What is Woman? Disease," to Freud who contended that women were inferior creatures suffering from penis envy, castration complexes, and a host of neuroses, the unique physiology and psychology of women have largely been misunderstood. This has frequently led to surgical excesses, especially during the nineteenth century. Dr. J. Marion Sims, a prominent name in gynecology even to this day, operated repeatedly on slave women, without the use of anesthesia and without their consent, to perfect his cure for vesicovaginal fistula, which is an abnormal pathway between the bladder and vagina that usually occurs as a result of birth trauma. Others performed clitoridectomies as a "cure" for nymphomania and masturbation. (Female circumcision is still performed on millions of young girls in many parts of the world.) However, the ovary took the greatest abuse.

In *Understanding Hysterectomy*, Drs. Giustini and Keefer recount the story of a "daring young doctor," Kentucky surgeon Dr. Ephraim McDowell, who in 1809, "without the benefit of anesthesia and sterile technique," is credited with performing the first oophorectomy, removing an ovarian tumor in a middle-aged woman. One has to wonder exactly who was the "daring" one—the doctor or the patient! But the onslaught was not to begin in earnest for another forty years when dentist William T. G. Morton demonstrated the use of ether to anesthetize a patient. Now that women could be put to sleep, it became open season on the female internal organs. From the middle or late 1800s until as recently as the 1940s, thousands of women had their ovaries sacrificed, frequently for trivial and irrelevant reasons such as overeating, disagreeable personalities, or lustful tendencies, and frequently at the cost of their lives. Martin Pernick, in *A Calculus of Suffering*, estimates that prior to 1846 (the year anesthesia was introduced by Morton), perhaps a hundred oophorectomies had been performed throughout the history of medicine. From 1846 to 1878, a single physician, Dr. William Atlee, took out the ovaries of nearly four hundred women. The champion of the oophorectomy movement was Robert Battey, a surgeon from Georgia who believed that through removal of the ovaries, one could control a woman's personality. Like Battey, Dr. David Gilliam boasted that after oophorectomy, his patients were "tractable, orderly, industrious and cleanly." When some of their colleagues, such as Elizabeth Blackwell, America's first female doctor, balked, these gynecologists argued that insane women—who were, of course, insane because they had wayward ovaries—had, in the words of Dr. William Goodell, no defense against undergoing the surgery:

For, in the first place, an insane woman is no more a member of the body politic than a criminal; secondly, her death is always a relief to her dearest friends; thirdly, even in case of her recovery from mental disease, she is liable to transmit the taint of insanity to her children and to her children's children for many generations. . . .

Because the uterus seemed in the minds of these male surgeons to be more directly linked to a woman's ability to bear children than were her ovaries, the battle to make the removal of the uterus commonplace was longer and more difficult than the fight for the oophorectomy. Ultimately, however, hysterectomy took root as the solution for that evil curse of the female form: menstruation. From earliest times, philosophers such as Aristotle and Pliny the Elder warned of menstruating women: that they could cause wine to sour and crops to die; that their very look could bewitch an innocent person. And of course the word "hysteria" comes to us from the Greek term for uterus because it was believed that insanity derived from a "wandering" of this organ. Menstruation was thought of as a monthly bloodletting whereby the body would rid itself of its poisons and excrements, automatically rendering women weak and inferior creatures. In 1868 Jules Michelet said of menstruation, "In reality, fifteen or twenty days out of twenty-eight (we may say nearly always), woman is not only an invalid, but a wounded one. She ceaselessly suffers from love's eternal wound." Women were therefore obviously incapable of playing an equal role in society, and maybe, just maybe, they were even a little mad. (Vestiges of this are present today when events get blamed on premenstrual syndrome, or PMS.) Therefore, wouldn't a woman be "better off" without her uterus? Believe it or not, this notion lingers even today. The significant numbers of women who literally were being castrated over a century ago cannot begin to compare with the numbers today who suffer a similar fate as our enlightened civilization continues to practice hysterectomy and oophorectomy with astounding frequency.

THE MODERN DILEMMA

In the days when I first trained and began to practice as a gynecologist, both physicians and the general public viewed hysterectomy as a benign procedure—even as a welcome one. There is no question that statistics in 1965 regarding anesthesia, antibiotics, and blood replacement were certainly an improvement over those of the 1940s or even the 1950s. We had better monitoring devices and better analgesics, and the public, in general, viewed surgery as something that was restorative rather than destructive. Many women believed that they would be better off having their uterus removed: They wouldn't have to worry about the monthly menstrual bleeding, could avoid the concern of cancer, and could take hormones and be young and feminine forever. Medicine and science had finally solved most of their problems.

In *The Woman Patient*, Nancy Roeske cites a small study of women who had undergone hysterectomy in which she seems to imply that the procedure is a feminist's and career woman's dream—that these women no longer have to fear that either children or troublesome uteri will interfere with their jobs and hobbies. The author of the study goes on to admit, however, that these women experienced fatigue, constipation, gastritis, hot flashes, insomnia, and "mourning" for up to a year postoperatively, but that these symptoms were "*not incapacitating*" [emphasis added].

Even more dramatic are the statements made in *Novak's Textbook of Gynecology* (Novak et al., 1975) calling the uterus a "worthless organ" once childbearing is completed, and best eliminated because worse than being worthless, the uterus was the source of the menses. The authors wrote that "menstruation is a nuisance to most women, and if this can be abolished . . . it would probably be a blessing to not only the women *but to their husbands* [emphasis added] . . ."

Giustini and Keefer in *Understanding Hysterectomy* take this mindset one step further, making it clear that under no circumstances should one hesitate to perform a hysterectomy on a postmenopausal woman, whether menopause had occurred naturally or had been accomplished surgically:

> She is no longer capable of becoming pregnant. The life-giving function of the uterus and ovaries has stopped. From this point on, there is no known value or function of the uterus. The ovaries, on the other hand, continue to function with decreasing hormone production, a fact that is considered by most American gynecologists to be of little value to the patient from a standpoint of good health and well being. . . .

> It is well accepted that when both ovaries are removed the uterus should be removed; only in exceptional circumstances should this organ be left in. The reason is a simple one—when both ovaries have been removed, the uterus becomes a functionless organ. The patient will not menstruate through it, and she will not be able to bear children with it. When one considers the risk of developing cancer in this now useless organ, it is obvious why it is best removed.

I recall a case in which a woman in her twenties had to have an ovary removed because of endometriosis (a buildup of abnormal tissue on the pelvic organs and in the abdominal cavity; see Chapter 4). When she first consulted with me, her other ovary was also severely involved. After two laparoscopic surgeries to attempt to save her remaining ovary (and hence her fertility), she finally had to have it removed because of disabling pain. I preserved her uterus and started her on estrogen replacement therapy. Today, that woman could have become pregnant with donor eggs and the advances of assisted reproductive technology. This story illustrates that it is never wise to remove healthy organs simply because they appear to be "useless."

The uterus and ovaries continue to be vital to women beyond childbearing, beyond menopause, and beyond their purely reproductive functions. But this view was not so widely held in the mid-1960s. Rather, the fear of cancer was overwhelming. Unfortunately, physicians capitalized, perhaps unwittingly, on this all-pervasive fear. Small fibroid tumors were considered potentially dangerous, and literally millions of hysterectomies were performed over the last twenty years with the diagnosis of rapidly enlarging fibroid tumors. Many of these tumors had grown from walnut to plum size and were the rationale for the hysterectomy. Uterine relaxation, or prolapse, was one of the frequent diagnoses used to justify hysterectomy, and with patients increasingly being covered by health insurance, surgery was now more affordable than ever. Another impetus to the growing number of hysterectomies was the sterilization committee that ruled on the proper requirements for sterilization. Depending on the patient's age, she might be required to have as many as four, five, or even six children before she would pass the criteria to be allowed sterilization. And remember, it was not until 1965 that the birth control pill came into general use, and of course abortion was illegal, so sterilization was a significant method of contraception in the 1950s and early 1960s.

Historically, many physicians circumvented these rules by performing hysterectomies. In 1975 the American College of Obstetricians and Gynecologists estimated that 20 percent of hysterectomies were performed solely for sterilization purposes. Nationwide, hysterectomy rates rose precipitously.

Certain physicians didn't even draw the line at sterilization on demand by women. These physicians might determine sterilization to be "necessary" in certain extenuating circumstances, such as mental retardation. Again, we quote from Giustini and Keefer:

> A menstrual period can be a very traumatic event for a mentally
> retarded female. She does not understand the blood loss and she

may not be able to cope with it. Also, the mentally retarded child can easily be the victim of unscrupulous sex offenders. A consequent pregnancy is an extremely serious situation.

One can only imagine how Giustini and Keefer would rate the physical and emotional trauma of major abdominal surgery (with the fear of hospitalization and the associated postoperative pain during the six-week recovery period) compared with the "trauma" of menses. Nor can one comprehend how having a hysterectomy prevents or even minimizes sexual abuse.

Be that as it may, surgeons often felt they were doing women a favor by justifying to the tissue committees (committees in hospitals that review pathology specimens—such as organs removed during surgery—to assure that normal, healthy tissue is not being removed unnecessarily) the indications for hysterectomy. My colleagues were well aware that the procedures were being done for sterilization, and I can personally recall numerous incidents when I offered women the opportunity to have a hysterectomy for sterilization, under the guise of uterine relaxation, vaginal prolapse, or recurrent abdominal bleeding. When I look back over those days, I realize that even though we were trying to help our patients, in the long run we probably did more harm than good.

I can vividly remember a patient who in 1970, only a few years after I had entered practice, desperately desired sterilization. She had two children and a history of irregular vaginal bleeding. On examination, I noted that she also had some uterine relaxation. I offered her a vaginal hysterectomy and vaginal tightening. The vaginal tissues were cinched, the uterus was removed, and the bladder was supported. The surgical procedure went quickly and smoothly, with no apparent problems. Shortly after we entered the recovery room, however, I noted that the patient was breathing with significant difficulty and small bubbles of fluid were coming out of her mouth. I listened to her chest and immediately made the diagnosis of pulmonary edema (fluid in the lungs), usually a result of heart failure and probably brought on by poor oxygen supply during surgery. This perfectly healthy forty-year-old woman who entered the hospital for an elective surgical procedure was now at risk for her life. We took emergency measures, which included placing a tube in her trachea (windpipe) and giving her oxygen, drugs to strengthen the force of her heart, and diuretics to relieve any fluid overload. She lived.

I remember turning away from her after the emergency measures were undertaken and saying to myself, "What a close call." It was then I began to ask, "Was this worth it?" Was it worth exposing this woman to mortal danger for a procedure that was not absolutely necessary? Fortunately, anesthesia is much improved today. We have constant oxygen monitoring; we intubate all patients during major surgery. Nevertheless, one hears of sporadic episodes of healthy young men and woman entering the hospital for a "benign" surgical condition and then dying of complications. I always think to myself the common bromide, the best safety device is a careful driver. Maybe the best safety device is to have surgery only when you must.

As I look back over those traumatic days, one point keeps pounding at me repeatedly: I don't think we physicians were ever totally imbued with the awesome responsibility that we had to protect our patients. I certainly was never adequately impressed by what it meant to be responsible for someone's life.

I knew one physician who set her own standards for medicine—standards perhaps one level above everyone else with whom I came in contact: Dr. Sophia Kleegman. A pioneer in her own right, Dr. Kleegman deserves a great deal of credit for sowing the seeds of doubt in my mind about the wisdom of the procedures that we performed. She was kind; she related to me as a physician; and I spent a lot of time following her around the clinics at Bellevue, learning from her insights and appreciating her compassion and sensitivity for her patients. She became a reproductive specialist when that was a rarity. Many of the residents did not take her seriously because she was so kind and homey; however, her patients took her very seriously. Other gynecologists would send her patients with a chronic vaginal infection called trichomonas, because she would spend a great deal of time instructing them on hygiene and trying to help them overcome this problem. Today we have a very specialized antibiotic, Flagyl, that eliminates these infections in one to two days; but Dr. Kleegman taught me never to give up on a patient and to make every effort to deal with her problem. She also showed me that the standard approach to a medical problem is not always the correct one.

Dr. Kleegman was really the first teacher to show me that just practicing expectant observation, what some call "doing nothing," can be the best medicine for some patients. She had a very large practice and many of her patients had fibroid tumors, but often she would just examine and monitor and not operate. Many of the young physicians jokingly referred to these patients as Dr. Kleegman's garden of fibroids. Most other physicians would have done hysterectomies and profited greatly from this garden, but Dr. Kleegman was different. She merely treated these patients with tender loving care, saw them once every six months to a year, and as long as their symptoms were not terribly significant, she kept them from the clutches of the surgeon.

I must admit that I did not always follow Dr. Kleegman's dictum of expectant observation. It was certainly easy to get on the bandwagon to perform the surgical procedure that we were taught was "our operation" and to start thinking about how many hysterectomies we could do. Over the years, both the trauma that my patients have faced and my own introspection have gradually taught me to appreciate the wisdom of her thinking, and to finally come to the realization that sometimes the best thing we can do for a patient is to do nothing.

One of my real bêtes noires is the terms "indicated" versus "necessary." In the old days we used to justify hysterectomy by citing "indications," such as a growing fibroid or recurrent vaginal bleeding. Whether these symptoms were excessive or not, whether it was the last straw or not, we tried to convince our patients that hysterectomy was the best option that could solve the problem—we could cut out the disease. There would be no change in their bodies or minds; they would only be healthier for what we were able to do for them! We began to believe our own hype that the presence of this tumor was some evil situation best resolved by removing the uterus. Why would anyone want to leave a fibroid uterus in a woman in her forties when the tumor (and the uterus) could be removed? We were all wrong. How could we have known that this mind-set would cost lives, lead to unnecessary suffering and pain, and not really improve the quality of most patients' lives? Therefore, when you hear "The surgery is indicated," remember to ask if it is indicated or it is necessary.

I now strongly believe that surgery should not be performed unless it will significantly improve the quality of the patient's life, unless it is the only proper course of action, and unless the alternatives require that it be performed. For example, ovarian tumors are potentially dangerous; they are often silent killers. No responsible physician would leave a persistent ovarian tumor and not recommend surgery. Cancer of the uterus or cervix is also a potentially lethal condition if untreated.

However, 99.8 percent of fibroids are benign. They are not potentially lethal. In these cases, I believe that the doctor and the patient should do all in their power to avoid the radical approach of hysterectomy, with its attendant complications and its psychological destructiveness. Saving or greatly improving the quality of a woman's life is the only true indication for surgery.

INDICATED OR NECESSARY?

Although it probably began in the 1940s, the debate concerning necessary versus unnecessary hysterectomy didn't really heat up until about twenty years ago when certain physicians and researchers began to notice some very disturbing trends in the statistics on hysterectomy. The most basic and alarming of these was the escalation in the numbers of procedures being performed. From 1965 to 1975, the annual number of hysterectomies in the United States had spiraled upward from 427,000 to 725,000. Women now had about a 62 percent chance that they would undergo hysterectomy. Like a cancer, surgical procedures were multiplying at a rate that was four times the growth rate of the population.

Of crucial interest to these researchers was that the growing numbers of hysterectomies were totally unrelated to any coinciding growth in the amount of pathology in women; in other words, women weren't any more diseased than before. So what was the cause of all of these hysterectomies?

Writing in the *New England Journal of Medicine* in 1979, Dr. John Bunker exposed some astonishing new data. The United States had twice as many surgeons in proportion to the overall population as did England and Wales, and U.S. surgeons performed twice as many operations. Hysterectomy was specifically shown to be even more excessive, with relative rates of 213 per 100,000 in the British Isles compared with 516 per 100,000 in the United States. Bunker cited "socioeconomic, organizational, philosophical, geographical, and population differences," but could find no medical reasons to account for the discrepancy. In other words, according to Bunker, the British system of socialized medicine had inherent safeguards and lacked incentives for surgery that differed from the American fee-for-service system. The safeguard is the "hourglass." In other words, a doctor can perform only a set number of surgeries in any given day; thus, if there are fewer doctors, there has to be less surgery. Today, the United Kingdom has approximately 1,000 OB-GYN specialists for a population of 25 million women. The United States has 30,000 such specialists for 125 million women—that's six times as many specialists per patient!

By the 1970s many Americans had health insurance plans that allowed them to afford the "luxury" of "elective" surgery. They could simply go to their doctor, sometimes a general practitioner, who would recommend and perform an operation without a second opinion being called for. In England, however, surgeons practiced out of hospitals, not in solo settings, and relied on referrals from general practitioners or internists to build their caseload. Rather than being gatekeepers they were consultants—the end of the line. And socialized medicine offered no financial gain in doing vast numbers of operations.

Finally, according to Bunker, there seemed to be a fundamental philosophical difference between the U.S. surgeon's attitude toward what operating could accomplish and the British surgeon's attitude. American doctors, said Bunker, were "more aggressive" and held "higher expectations." That

American doctors derive great satisfaction from performing surgery seems to be supported by the research done by Diane Scully. She interviewed obstetrician-gynecologists in training at New England hospitals. Nothing can illustrate the attitudes of eager new surgeons better than this passage from her interview with one young doctor:

> You open the belly . . . you take something out, and the patient gets better . . . I don't know, it is the same thing as in kindergarten when you took a little car apart. . . . The thing with surgery is that you have something to show. You have a headache and I give you an aspirin and it goes away, fine. If you have postpartum bleeding and you need a hysterectomy and I take out your uterus and everything is fine, you can say, "Look at that fine piece of surgery I did."

How doctors are educated and the philosophies instilled in them by the standards of the community where they practice seem to play key roles in how they approach surgery. Consider the results of an extensive study published in *Scientific American* by John Wennberg and Alan Gittelsohn a few years after Bunker's. Surprisingly, the authors found that "the amount and cost of hospital treatment [including surgery] in a community have more to do with the numbers of physicians there, their medical specialties, and the procedures they prefer than with the health of the residents." They discussed an almost unbelievable example of two cities in Maine less than twenty miles apart. In the first city, hysterectomy was done so frequently that if the rate were to persist, 70 percent of the women there would have had a hysterectomy by the time they were seventy years old! In the second city, only 25 percent would have. In examining the health of the two groups of women residing in each city, they found no differences. Neither could they explain this phenomenon by citing a difference in wealth, insurance coverage, or even the numbers of physicians or hospital beds. It seemed the sole difference between these two communities was in the style of medical practice—one city's doctors were "enthusiastic" about hysterectomy, while the other's were "skeptical of its value." The residents in communities with wide disparities between surgical rates still seemed to perceive themselves as having an equal level of health and well-being. In addition, those with the less aggressive surgeons did not seek their operations elsewhere. More recent studies confirm that these factors are still with us in the 1990s. In 1996 a study published in the journal *Health Services Research* revealed that physician factors, including background characteristics and training, experience, and practice style, played a "statistically significant role in the hysterectomy decision" in one analysis of 36,104 cases performed by 339 doctors in 43 hospitals in Arizona.

Additional interesting and disturbing trends were provided by Richard Dicker and his associates in the *Journal of the American Medical Association (JAMA)* in 1982. Hysterectomy, it seemed, was a much more likely scenario for you if you were black or from the South. Even as the overall numbers of operations declined from the late 1970s into the 1980s and now have stabilized, Southern women continue to undergo the most hysterectomies and at the youngest age. (The rate in the Northeast is the lowest in the nation.)

Over a decade after that *JAMA* article, Kristen Kjerulff et al. reported in a 1993 issue of *Obstetrics and Gynecology* that the average annual age-adjusted hysterectomy rate was still higher for black women than for white women (49.5 per 10,000 for black women versus 41.2 per 10,000 for white women). The study, which looked at more than 53,000 hysterectomies performed in Maryland between 1986 and 1991, also revealed that black women were more than twice as likely to be diagnosed with uterine fibroids—a condition frequently successfully treated with much less radical techniques (see Chapter 3). The worst news from this study was that black women were more likely to suffer complications, have a longer hospitalization, and had *three times the in-hospital death rate as that of white women.* Furthermore, the authors could offer no explanations, citing that "It is not clear why black women having hysterectomy in this study were at higher risk than white women for complications, extended hospitalizations and mortality."

A smaller study by Kjerulff et al., published in the *American Journal of Public Health* in 1993, examined socioeconomic factors (including education, income, and race) in 12,465 women and did not find race to be a factor. Instead, they discovered that in the United States, women with less education and lower incomes are more likely to undergo hysterectomy. (Other studies confirm that this is also true globally.)

Interestingly, if surgeons know that they are being monitored, it has a profound effect on how frequently they perform this procedure. In 1977, Frank Dyck and his associates published a now famous study in the *New England Journal of Medicine*: The health department in Saskatchewan, Canada, had noted a 72 percent increase in the number of hysterectomies between 1964 and 1971. Growing concerned, the department appointed a committee to keep watch on the overall number and underlying diagnoses of hysterectomies. The committee compiled a list of indications for hysterectomy, and then analyzed each procedure to see whether it was indicated according to the established criteria. It found that in the seven hospitals it examined over a four-year period, "the average proportion of unjustified hysterectomies had dropped from 23.7 percent at the time of the first review to 7.8 percent. . . . The total number of hysterectomies in the province dropped by 32.8 percent." The authors were encouraged by the results, but expressed regret that such a committee had ever been necessary.

Similarly, seeking second opinions for hysterectomy often has an effect on performance rates, but only in certain geographic regions. In 1990 the journal *Medical Care* published a report by Madelon Finkel and David Finkel of 1,698 women referred by their insurance company for a mandatory second opinion prior to getting a hysterectomy. One hundred thirty-five of these women were advised on second opinion not to have the surgery. Women in the Northeast tended not to have the operation when it was not confirmed on second opinion. By contrast, women from the South and Midwest went through with surgery even when not confirmed on second opinion and even when, as the authors put it, "some hysterectomies were performed for questionable reasons, i.e., symptoms did not warrant surgical intervention, no pathologic justification, or conservative treatment preferable."

Last, but certainly not least, we discover some fascinating facts concerning hysterectomies and physicians themselves. For instance, doctors' wives were found to have an even higher rate of hysterectomy than the general female population. This might lead us to believe, therefore, that physicians truly had confidence in what they were doing, and were not performing unnecessary surgery for ulterior motives, such as monetary rewards. However, female gynecologists have much lower hysterectomy rates than do wives of male gynecologists.

In addition, gender may play a role. As recently as 1994, epidemiologists discovered that male gynecologists who are older and therefore further from their training, and who practice in remote areas that have small numbers of gynecologists, perform more hysterectomies. This study by Nina Bickell et al., published in the *American Journal of Public Health*, found that *male doctors performed 60 percent more hysterectomies than female physicians*, but it was unclear if this was because of their sex or because their training had not been as recent. They also found that appropriateness ratings were affected by both patient's and doctor's attitudes toward surgery. They suggest that "To decrease their chances of undergoing hysterectomy, patients should express their preferences [desire to avoid surgery]. . . ." (And that is exactly what this book is all about.)

We have seen that hysterectomy is a very controversial operation—the "necessity" and frequency of which seem to vary according to who you are, who your doctor is, and where you live even more than what your diagnosis is. When hysterectomies first came under intense scrutiny, no re-searcher could definitively state whether the discrepancies repeatedly found from country to country and across various regions of the United States meant too much surgery in one place or too little surgery in another. To attempt to answer this controversy, doctors began to analyze the risks and benefits, the morbidity and mortality rates, and to come up with guide-lines, or indications, for hysterectomy.

To understand this, first we have to take a look at why hysterectomies were (and still are) being done. Contrary to what most people might be-lieve, cancer is the underlying reason for uterine removal only 11 percent of the time. Fibroids account for a significant portion of all hysterectomies: about 34 percent. Roughly 16 percent are performed to correct a relaxation of the pelvic structures that has allowed the uterus to prolapse. En-dometriosis (when pieces of the uterine lining implant on structures outside the uterus) is the diagnosis in nearly 20 percent of cases. (Endometriosis is the only diagnosis for which the numbers of hysterectomies have increased instead of decreased—up from the 15 percent mentioned in the first edition of this book.) A small number of hysterectomies (approximately 20 percent) seem to be performed for a variety of very rare conditions, such as obstet-rical emergencies and severe infections (see Table 1.1).

Of greatest concern and controversy, however, were (and still are) hysterectomies that are performed for so-called cancer prevention and ster-ilization. According to Naomi Miller Stokes in *The Castrated Woman*, 27 percent of all American women are unable to have children, largely be-cause of hysterectomy. We need only go back a decade or two to discover

Table 1.1 Reasons for Hysterectomies, 1988–1990

Diagnosis	Percentage of total hysterectomies	Rate per 10,000 women
Fibroids	33.5	19.0
Endometriosis	18.2	10.3
Prolapse	16.2	9.2
Cancer	11.2	6.3
Endometrial hyperplasia	6.0	3.4
Menstrual/menopausal symptoms	4.5	2.6
Cervical dysplasia	1.4	0.8
Pain	0.6	0.3
Other	8.5	4.8

Adapted from Lynne Wilcox, et al., "Hysterectomy in the United States, 1988–1990." *Obstetrics and Gynecology* 83, no. 4 (April 1994): 552.

some horrifying facts: From Ann Arbor, Michigan, where 68.5 percent of all vaginal hysterectomies were performed for "socioeconomic" and "multiparity" reasons, to Los Angeles, where elective hysterectomy rates for sterilization rose in one hospital by 742 percent in two years, the overall rate of sterilization by hysterectomy increased by 293 percent between 1968 and 1970! This was particularly troubling because bilateral tubal ligation, a much simpler and safer procedure accomplishing sterilization, was common knowledge.

Perhaps the reason for the switch from minor surgery (tubal ligation) to major surgery (hysterectomy) can be explained by a fad of so-called prophylactic, or preventative, hysterectomies. In the early 1970s, one gynecologist declared to his colleagues that the time had come for them to "recognize and recommend prophylactic elective total hysterectomy and bilateral salpingooophorectomy [removal of both fallopian tubes and ovaries] as . . . proper preventative medicine in obstetrics and gynecology." (One wonders what he would have thought of a urologist who might have recommended to him that his prostate be removed as "proper preventative medicine" because 60 percent of males over age sixty develop prostate cancer. The potential complications of this surgery, including urinary incontinence and impotence, make routine prostatectomy unthinkable.) This was not an extreme opinion of an eccentric gynecologist. The American College of Obstetrics and Gynecologists debated the controversy of elective hysterectomy at a meeting in 1971. In the end, supporters of the procedure significantly outclapped opponents, as measured on an audiometer. Dr. James H. Sammons, executive vice president of the American Medical Association, sided with the majority. In 1977 he concurred that elective hysterectomies as a "convenient form of sterilization and . . . their prophylactic use to eliminate the possibility of uterine cancer in future years" was legitimate. While it might not be necessary in either case, he argued that it was "beneficial to women with excessive anxiety."

Fortunately, as we shall soon see, society did not agree that hysterectomy was such a bargain. Feminists, congressional representatives, and insurance companies, among others, began to erode these ideas. They were alarmed that of the half million women having hysterectomies each year, approximately 2,000 would die, another 200,000 would suffer nonfatal complications, and over 100,000 would require blood transfusions. This was exclusive of the millions of health care dollars expended on potentially unnecessary hysterectomies, not to mention time lost from employment or child-care duties.

Shocking revelations of surgical abuse came from all corners of society. For example, in a 1976 audit Blue Cross/Blue Shield discovered that as many as 40 percent of hysterectomies performed in certain parts of the country resulted in the removal of totally normal organs for cancer or pregnancy prevention. As a result, during the mid to late 1970s, insurance companies began to require patients to obtain a second opinion before undergoing major surgery.

Congress investigated this matter in 1976 and reported in "Cost and Quality of Health Care" that hysterectomy was "questionable in 40 percent of cases including when it was done for obsessive fear of pregnancy and acute cancerphobia." The media had a field day reporting on unnecessary operations and quoting doctors who candidly admitted that out came "a uterus or two each month to pay the rent." Of course, where doctors are concerned, lawyers are soon to follow. On the subject of medical malpractice, David Louisell and Harold Williams wrote, "Foremost among . . . surgical operations [performed without reasonable indications] are various gynecologic procedures."

If sterilization and cancer prevention did not justify hysterectomy, then what did? What were the valid "medical indications" for removal of the uterus? The response to this question came from many circles, primarily physicians and quality assurance committees.

Writing in a 1976 issue of the *New England Journal of Medicine*, gynecologist Valentina Clark Donahue declared the following to be "the appropriate indications for hysterectomy":

- Premalignant states and localized invasive cancers of the cervix, endometrium, ovaries or fallopian tubes
- Symptomatic nonmalignant conditions of the uterus [such as fibroids] compressing adjacent pelvic structures and giving rise to repeated uterine bleeding not responsive to curettage [D&C]
- Uterine bleeding not responsive to hormonal therapy, or uterine pain or bleeding in women in whom hormonal therapy is contraindicated, such as in women with adenomyosis [a condition whereby the lining of the endometrium grows inward, invading the muscle lining of the uterus]
- Diseases of the tubes and ovaries in which the uterus is not primarily involved but removed as part of the extirpation of these diseased adnexal appendages [pelvic organs] (e.g., chronic advanced tubal infections or severe endometriosis with extensive scarring of genital structures)
- Symptomatic descent or prolapse of the uterus caused by disease or derangement of supporting structures
- Removal of the uterus necessitated by operations for primary neoplasia [cancer] of adjacent structures

- Obstetric catastrophes, including uncontrollable bleeding or uterine rupture
- Therapeutic abortion in the first trimester [three months] of gestation [pregnancy] in selected cases for multiparous women [women with more than one child] who desire sterilization and for whom other forms of fertility control are contraindicated or not desired
- Septic abortion [abortion resulting in uterine infection] not responsive to curettage [D&C] and medical therapy

In 1977, the American College of Obstetricians and Gynecologists issued a policy statement that ranked gynecological surgery in order of necessity. So-called emergency situations would include hemorrhage of a tubal pregnancy, for example. Next in line were "mandatory" operations for "the presence of a malignancy." This was followed by "urgent" situations including "abnormal uterine bleeding which requires further diagnostic evaluation or definitive treatment." Then there were conditions for which surgery is "advisable," such as prolapse, and finally "elective" procedures for "family planning purposes."

The Professional Standards and Review Organization (PSRO), a hospital watchdog group responsible for auditing hospital stays and monitoring quality of care, agreed with only four of the above "medically appropriate indications for hysterectomy": cancer and premalignant diseases, fibroids, abnormal bleeding conditions, and prolapsed uterus.

In a 1993 review article in the *New England Journal of Medicine*, Dr. Karen Carlson and her colleagues updated the indications for hysterectomy. They noted that "professional uncertainty about the appropriate use of hysterectomy is the primary cause of the variation in rates [of hysterectomy in different parts of the United States and the world]. . . . The uncertainty is thought to stem from difficulties in diagnosis, lack of information on the probable outcomes of hysterectomy and alternative treatments, and differences between physicians' judgments and patients' preferences for treatment." These authors still maintained most of Dr. Donahue's now twenty-year-old indications, but with certain caveats. For example, with respect to cancer, no longer is hysterectomy indicated as a blanket treatment for "premalignant states and localized invasive cancers of the cervix or endometrium." However, they maintain that "Initial hysterectomy is indicated for atypical hyperplasia (a premalignant state of the lining of the uterus; see Chapter 6) when the patient desires a definitive procedure or is postmenopausal."

Carlson also noted that fibroids still account for about one-third of all hysterectomy procedures and was critical of the practice when patients did not have any symptoms. She and her colleagues pointed out that fibroids generally stabilize or shrink after menopause and that there has been no proof of the argument that there is increased operative risk to a woman if her fibroids are allowed to remain and possibly enlarge should she need surgery (on potentially larger fibroids) later. Furthermore, they discounted another reason traditionally "sold" to patients—that even though they are experiencing no symptoms now, they could avoid symptoms in the future by having their fibroids removed: "Predicting which patients will have symptoms is difficult . . . and there is no evidence to support this rationale for hysterectomy." In other words, don't bother it if it's not bothering you.

Carlson and her colleagues continue to support the traditional indications for hysterectomy, including symptomatic fibroids, abnormal uterine bleeding, uterine prolapse, endometriosis, adenomyosis, chronic pelvic pain, pelvic infections, malignant and certain premalignant conditions of the reproductive organs, and pregnancy-related emergencies. Within almost every category, however, they qualify these indications with information about alternatives to hysterectomy that should be attempted prior to resorting to this radical surgery. They conclude that "Current indications for hysterectomy have evolved considerably from the time when sterilization, fear of cancer, and undiagnosed pelvic pain were common reasons for the procedure." But they note that no clear consensus exists on when hysterectomy should be favored over alternative treatments for "benign" conditions, because there is not enough data comparing outcomes of hysterectomy versus other management techniques for the same conditions.

As a result of this lack of clear information, even the experts can't agree. Nina Bickell and her associates published a study in the *American Journal of Public Health* in 1995 that compared ratings of the "appropriateness of hysterectomy" between a national panel of experts and practicing community gynecologists. They discovered a distinct difference of opinion regarding appropriateness within both the expert group and the community group, and thus concluded, "For areas of clinical uncertainty in which experts' opinions are used in guideline development, additional measures such as process of care, quality of life, and patient preferences should be included in discussions about guidelines."

I couldn't agree more with the authors of this study. I believe that many of the above indications, stated first by Dr. Donahue and then by Dr. Carlson, are poor reasons for hysterectomy and represent a skewed and outdated mentality now that alternative modes of treatment exist. In the following chapters, I will explain why. Yet, you can open any textbook today and still see some variation of these "medical indications" for hysterectomy.

The next logical question is, what if a hysterectomy is described to you as "indicated"? Does that mean you will be happier for it, will benefit from it, that it will improve the quality of your existence? Will it be worth risking your life? Can the health care system budget tolerate surgery done for mere comfort and convenience? With the exception of the recent intolerance for spiraling health care costs, the jury is still out on these questions, despite numerous studies to attempt to answer them.

In a 1985 issue of *Medical Care*, Sonia Sandberg and her colleagues analyzed elective hysterectomies. They found that if a woman having her uterus removed for a benign process is destined to develop cancer (a very small minority), then her life expectancy will increase by roughly six to eight years. However, for the majority—who do not develop cancer, but who would then be at increased risk of heart disease from having either a decline or cessation of ovarian function—there would be a *decreased* life expectancy. And obviously for those unfortunate women who die from the surgery, an average of over thirty-nine years of life would be stolen from them.

Overall, Sandberg and her colleagues were of the opinion that elective hysterectomy did increase the quality of one's life. However, because it couldn't be predicted how women would perceive their inability to bear children (to some it would be an advantage; to others a disadvantage) or what psychological impact the removal of the uterus would have, these very significant factors were omitted from the study. In my opinion, these omissions are significant and may have altered the authors' interpretation of the data concerning quality of life.

Harvard physician and epidemiologist Dr. Philip Cole studied the same question. He also found that a thirty-five-year-old woman having an elective hysterectomy would benefit from an increased life expectancy, relief of some symptoms such as irregular uterine bleeding, and economic gains. However, 98.7 percent of the female population would not contract uterine cancer and would therefore expect no increase in their life expectancy. The overall 0.2 year increase in life expectancy (a statistical average) was exactly the same as the amount of time the average woman spends recovering from a hysterectomy! Furthermore, each year of life saved in the name of cancer prevention would be costly, and the years gained would be lived during old age—probably after age seventy-five. Finally, the economic gains to society from the elimination of Pap smears, obstetrical care, D&Cs, contraceptives, and so forth for the women undergoing hysterectomy would be exceeded by its costs to the tune of $1.5 billion! In conclusion, said Dr.

Cole, "Cancer prophylaxis cannot justify elective hysterectomy . . . the gains are uncertain but small and the potential health losses are great. We cannot assess the value of hysterectomy for contraception or other quality-of-life reasons, such as to reduce fear of cancer or to eliminate frequent, unpredictable bleeding."

Everyone agrees that hysterectomy can lead to complications, the specifics of which we describe in a later chapter. However, the cruel irony in all of this is that after numerous studies, meetings, and position papers, doctors remain embroiled in a bitter controversy regarding indicated versus necessary hysterectomies. This controversy strikes at the very livelihood of the obstetrician-gynecologist—his or her reason for existence. Old habits die hard, and no two doctors will give you exactly the same answer on this issue.

My opinion is that just because a condition may be a legitimate indication for surgery doesn't really mean that that condition *necessitates* surgery. For example, suppose a forty-year-old woman has a large fibroid, but she is unaware of its presence. It causes her absolutely no pain or excessive bleeding. Why subject this woman to the perils and discomforts of a hysterectomy? Unfortunately, the average woman attended by the average gynecologist will be "sold" a hysterectomy. She will be subtly convinced that her enlarging uterus might be an ominous precursor to cancer. With hysterectomy, the doctor will argue, she will be spared not only from this potential cancer but from her monthly menstrual inconvenience and any unwanted pregnancies. After all, hadn't Dr. Wright said in 1969 that after the last planned pregnancy the uterus becomes a "useless, bleeding, symptom producing, potentially cancer-bearing organ" that should be removed?

The truth is that doctors don't advocate hysterectomy because they are a bad lot; they do so because it is "their operation." When I was in medical school, the gynecology residents-in-training were so eager to do surgery that we literally had a sign posted in the gynecology exam room that read, "Donate your uterus." Hysterectomy was our universal solution to nearly any problem. Remember that doctors like to find solutions to problems because their patients demand solutions and because they truly derive satisfaction from helping people. And a typically American solution to a problem is not to fix it, but to throw it out—or maybe replace it with something newer and better, such as artificial hormones.

Between 1988 and 1990, the most recent years for which data is available, *1.7 million hysterectomies were performed in the United States.* One-third of women will undergo hysterectomy by age sixty-five—and most of these surgeries are elective! Today, hysterectomy is dying hard because younger doctors are still being trained by older, traditional-minded physicians. New equipment is expensive and difficult to master. Individual gynecologists don't appreciate the tremendous morbidity and mortality (the epidemiologists' terms for bad outcomes; in other words, serious complications including deaths) that hundreds of thousands of procedures a year add up to. Nor do conventional doctors think about the immediate impact on a woman in terms of her six or eight weeks of incapacitation and what that means to her in lost income and neglected family responsibilities. From the surgeon's perspective, a "pelvic house-cleaning" is very neat and tidy. They don't have to concern themselves with following a patient for future gynecologic problems. From the woman's perspective, she is entering a new era in her life, and she may not be prepared to cope with the loss she may experience in terms of her self-image as a complete woman. If there is any criticism that I have of the medical profession up to now, it is that we have treated the uterus rather than treating the patient.

That's the bad news. The good news is that this is changing. After peaking in 1975, hysterectomy rates gradually declined and now have plateaued at a rate of approximately 600,000 procedures per year since about 1988. Several factors may account for this change: Consumers of medical services are demanding change. As women became more savvy to the untoward effects of hysterectomy, they became less willing to succumb to the surgery. Technology is being developed every day to respond to the demand for more effective and less radical alternative treatments. The introduction of the birth control pill and the increased utilization of tubal sterilization and vasectomy also bring change.

Finally, for better or for worse, changes are also resulting from a new era of managed care. Patients and/or employers who foot the bill for health insurance and insurance companies themselves are forcing doctors and hospitals into mandated second opinions and into finding more efficient and more inexpensive ways of treating the traditional indications for hysterectomy. Managed care companies are tracking the proclivities of physicians to perform hysterectomies; as a result, physicians are now looking over their shoulders. The "indications" are tightening and will continue to make it harder for physicians who favor hysterectomy to have their way.

In 1989, perhaps driven by consumer demand and managed care, laparoscopic hysterectomy was introduced as a surgical tour de force and was subsequently modified and popularized as a laparoscopic-assisted vaginal hysterectomy (see Chapter 8). This technique, which allows the surgeon to convert an abdominal hysterectomy (a lengthy operation requiring a lengthy hospital stay) into a vaginal hysterectomy, is a definite advance *but* a feeding frenzy has developed to try to sell a "kinder, gentler hysterectomy." In actuality, the complication rate was initially very high because a learning curve is present in order for doctors to perform the operation successfully. In many places, this learning curve is still with us.

This concerns me because many women are sold a hysterectomy that gets them out of the hospital in one or two days and back to work in two weeks, but they still may not have needed that operation at all! Surgical advances such as these must be considered within the context of sound and conservative medical care.

Conversely, a recent book advocates myomectomy (removal of fibroids) instead of hysterectomy in *all* patients. I am wary of this approach as well. I have cared for many women who would not have been well served by myomectomy. Common sense dictates that a three-hour myomectomy surgery requiring the transfusion of three to four units of blood places a woman at much greater risk than a one-hour hysterectomy. The bottom line is that every woman is an individual and every situation is unique, requiring that the treatment plan—be it hysterectomy or a less radical approach—must be tailor-made to her specifications.

As you and your physician design your plan of care, you also have to take care not to be short-sighted about what doctors and researchers might discover in the future, which might make us regret the decision not to act in a minimally invasive manner. For example, consider this passage from a letter by Dr. Paul Stumpf published in a 1984 issue of the *Journal of the American Medical Association.* He wrote of the future of in vitro fertilization—pregnancies conceived in a "test tube" then transferred to the mother's womb:

> Successful pregnancies, in both monkey and human subjects without ovaries have been reported as a result of ovum transfer and simple hormonal replacement. This information suggests that the uterus may no longer be considered a useless organ in all women following oophorectomy, since subsequent pregnancy is now clearly a realistic technical possibility. For this reason, is [sic] seems appropriate to reexamine the advisability of the traditional incidental excision of an otherwise healthy uterus at surgery to remove the ovaries in young women who may nevertheless desire later childbearing.

Through advances in medical science, we now have an alternative to nearly every indication for hysterectomy. A prolapse may safely be left alone, unless it is really bothersome. In that case, reconstructive surgery can be performed to repair rather than remove the offending structures. Laparoscopic surgery offers hope for the woman with endometriosis or fibroids, for which there is also myomectomy (the surgical excision of uterine fibroids). Abnormal bleeding may be treated by hysteroscopic surgery or significantly reduced with hormonal therapy. Even certain precancerous lesions, depending on their location and the extent to which they have invaded the uterus, no longer mean automatic hysterectomy. The bottom line is that indicated hysterectomy does not equal necessary hysterectomy, as the following chapters will illustrate.

2

HOW YOUR REPRODUCTIVE SYSTEM NORMALLY WORKS

I really love getting my period. It's like the changing seasons. I feel a bond with other women. I feel fertile and womanly and empowered because of my potential to make a life. . . .
—The New Our Bodies, Ourselves

In the beginning, the fertilized embryo is female. It is only in the presence of the male sex hormone, testosterone, that the genital ridge near the fetal tail will differentiate into a male. The male is formed out of the female by an elongation of the embryonic clitoris into a penis. By the time a female fetus is a mere eight weeks old, she will have microscopic sex organs. The uterus and ovaries will be fully formed in six months. These organs play a key role in the overall normal physiologic functioning of a woman, which goes above and beyond the childbearing aspects. It is therefore essential that you understand the normal functioning of the female reproductive tract before going any further in our discussion on hysterectomy.

A normal newborn baby girl will have a clitoris and vagina, cervix and uterus, as well as two fallopian tubes and ovaries. Her ovaries will already contain an excess of 400,000 ova, or eggs—the only ones she will ever produce in her lifetime. (Her male counterpart, however, will continuously manufacture millions of sperm until he is well into his later years.) Once a month after puberty, she will release a single egg at ovulation. If sperm are present, the union of one sperm with the egg will result in the formation of a fertilized embryo, and the cycle will begin again for the next generation.

THE MENSTRUAL CYCLE AND YOUR CHANGING HORMONES

Every month, a woman undergoes a series of events brought about by a complex interaction among the nervous, endocrine, and reproductive systems of her body in preparation for a pregnancy. This is called the menstrual cycle. Day one of the menstrual cycle is marked by the first day of menstrual flow. Depending on the woman, bleeding may commence anywhere from every twenty to thirty-six days, and last from two to eight days. During this time, she will shed only about two to three tablespoons of blood, but it will be mixed with equal amounts of other secretions from the cervix, endometrium, and vagina. This bleeding is triggered by signals originating in the brain.

Deep within the midbrain is the hypothalamus, which is responsible for a variety of functions including telling us when we are hungry, thirsty, sleepy, hot, or cold. The hypothalamus is an endocrine gland; this means that it secretes hormones, which are chemical substances synthesized in one place, and then transported through the bloodstream to exert an effect on a distant organ of the body. Specifically, the hypothalamus secretes gonadotrophin releasing hormones (GnRH), which are then sent via a specially designed circulatory system to the pituitary gland, an area of the brain no larger than a pea. The pituitary gland is divided into two sections: One secretes hormones responsible for the uterine contractions that facilitate labor and delivery as well as the let down of milk in the breast-feeding mother; the other produces a host of chemicals regulating our growth and metabolism. It is this second portion of the gland that is stimulated by the hypothalamus to release its other major hormones, luteinizing hormone (LH) and follicle stimulating hormone (FSH) via the GnRH specific to each: LHRH and FSHRH, respectively. These then travel down to the ovary and trigger yet another round of activities, including the release of chemical substances. The ovary produces the female sex hormones estrogen and progesterone (called progestin in vivo), and a small amount of male sex hormones called androgens (principally testosterone). The ovary itself is composed of hundreds of thousands of clusters of cells containing immature eggs; these units are called follicles.

At the start of the menstrual cycle, estrogen and progesterone levels are at their lowest and thus exert a feedback effect on the hypothalamus, meaning that these depleted stores of estrogen and progesterone send a chemical message to the brain triggering the hypothalamus to release GnRH. The GnRH acts on the pituitary, which then releases large amounts of FSH with a small quantity of LH. The FSH (follicle stimulating hormone) then reaches the ovary where, as the name implies, it stimulates about a score of the immature follicles to mature. As they mature, the follicles produce estrogens that act on the endometrium, the mucous membrane lining the uterus. The endometrium thickens, thus producing a rich carpet of nutrients in preparation for the implantation of a fertilized egg. It will be the placenta, formed from the embryo, that supports a developing fetus should pregnancy occur. Because of this growth and thickening of the endometrium during this time, this phase of the menstrual cycle, roughly day six through thirteen, is called the proliferative phase.

FSH and LH levels continue to mount until one follicle breaks away from the pack and continues its development while the others simply wither. Within this follicle, the egg is undergoing a process whereby the genetic material is being packaged into twenty-three separate chromosomes, which will ultimately unite with twenty-three others provided by the male to produce the complete complement needed for a human being. The follicle increases its size five times over and migrates to the surface of the ovary where it will eventually burst and release its egg in the process called ovulation. (Theoretically, this occurs on day fourteen.)

The egg floats away from the ovary and is captured by the fingerlike projections on the end of the fallopian tube. Once within the tube, it will take approximately three to four days for the ovum to travel to the uterus. Swept along on its journey by tiny hairlike structures called cilia, it is here in the fallopian tube that fertilization can take place. The ovum continues along the tube until it reaches the uterus where it takes another three days to implant in the lining if fertilized, or pass out of the body unnoticed if not. (If, for reasons that are not understood, the egg implants in the fallopian tube instead of in the uterus, an ectopic pregnancy occurs. This is a potentially life-threatening situation if not detected early on, because as the embryo grows, it will stretch the tube beyond its limits until it eventually ruptures. This can cause the woman to bleed to death.)

Meanwhile, after the release of the egg, the ruptured follicle transforms itself into a specialized endocrine gland called the corpus luteum, or "yellow body," so named because the presence of cholesterol gives it this characteristic color. Rising levels of luteinizing hormone assure this transformation and cause the newly formed corpus luteum to produce estrogen and progesterone. This will maintain a pregnancy, should it occur, until the fetus is able to secrete its own hormones at about the eleventh week of pregnancy. Progesterone is the chemical that directs the endometrium to secrete nutrients for the developing fetus. Thus this phase is called the secretory (luteal) phase, and it lasts from about day fifteen to day twenty-eight in the cycle.

If an embryo is in the uterus, the placenta will produce a hormone known as human chorionic gonadotrophin (HCG). Chemically identical to LH, it takes over the role of the corpus luteum in stimulating estrogen and progesterone production. Pregnancy tests work on the principle of detecting rising levels of HCG as they are present only in pregnant women.

If no pregnancy has occurred, FSH and LH levels drop, the corpus luteum breaks down, and it no longer secretes progesterone and estrogen.

Without the support of these hormones, particularly progesterone, the uterine lining degenerates. Blood vessels shrink and rupture, depriving the tissue of needed nutrient support. A combination of blood and tissue now passes out of the uterus through its opening in the cervix in the process called menstruation. Low levels of estrogen and progesterone then feed back to the hypothalamus, beginning the process all over again (see Figure 2.1).

The average woman will go through approximately five hundred menstrual cycles in her life from menarche (the onset of menstruation) to menopause (the end of menstrual cycles). Before puberty, there is no gonadotrophic activity in either the hypothalamus or the pituitary and thus no ovarian activity. For reasons not clearly understood, estrogens keep the pituitary in check until about age eight. Thereafter, the pituitary begins to secrete increasing amounts of gonadotrophic hormones, which eventually lead up to the onset of menstrual periods.

During puberty, the transition into adulthood, the female reproductive organs mature and prepare themselves for their adult functions, including pregnancy, procreation, and breastfeeding. The female reproductive system is both internal and external (see Figures 2.2, 2.3, and 2.4). Breasts, vagina, and clitoris are external. At puberty, under the influence of increasing amounts of estrogens, the vagina enlarges and fat is deposited in the mons pubis and labia majora. Likewise, the labia minora and clitoris enlarge.

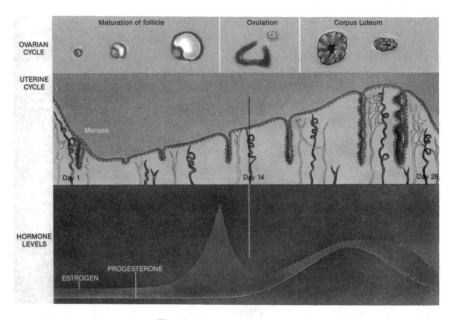

Figure 2.1 The menstrual cycle.

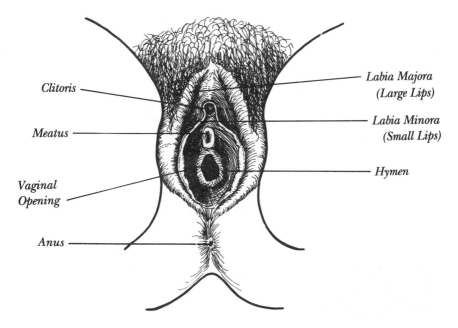

Clitoris

Meatus

Vaginal
Opening

Anus

Labia Majora
(Large Lips)

Labia Minora
(Small Lips)

Hymen

Figure 2.2 External female anatomy.

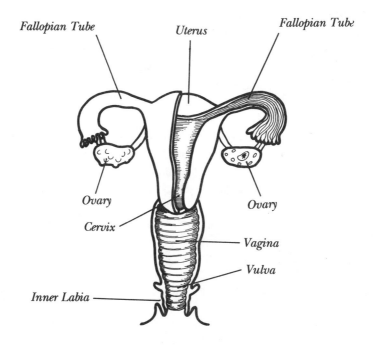

Fallopian Tube

Uterus

Fallopian Tube

Ovary

Cervix

Inner Labia

Ovary

Vagina

Vulva

Figure 2.3 Internal female anatomy, front view.

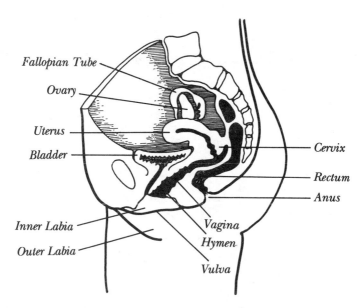

Figure 2.4 Internal female anatomy, side view.

Pubic hair begins to grow on the perineum. (Hair development seems to come from the influences of the male sex hormones, the androgens, rather than from estrogen.) Within the vagina, the cellular structures are changing as well. The cells that line the walls of the vagina, called the epithelium, change to a type that seems to be more resistant to trauma and infection.

The breasts also develop under the influences of estrogen: They grow larger, the nipples darken, and they initiate the development of the internal system of ducts and glands that will eventually produce milk for the newborn baby. However, the crucial completion of the milk-producing structures are under the influence of progesterone and prolactin. These hormones are produced by the ovary, placenta, and pituitary, respectively. In other words, while estrogens secreted during puberty lend the breasts their characteristically mature outward appearance, it is progesterone that is responsible for converting breasts to functioning organs.

If we imagine that we could look internally from a vantage point inside the vagina, the first thing that we would notice is a circular structure with an opening in the center. This is called the cervix, the "front door" to the uterus. In a woman who has never had children, the opening in the cervix (called the os) is small and round. If a woman has had children, the os is more elongated and may have an irregular shape from birth trauma. The cervix contains nerves and blood vessels that may play a role in female sexual response. Likewise, it produces a natural lubricant to increase comfort and pleasure during intercourse, to facilitate the passage of sperm into the uterus, and to provide a hostile environment for bacterial foreign invaders. The cervix comprises the lower third of the uterus, the three-layered muscular organ that houses the developing fetus.

Shaped like an upside-down pear, the uterus enlarges two- to threefold during puberty to about the size of a fist. Inside the uterus, estrogen-mediated changes are occurring in the lining. It is thickening and developing more glandular tissue. The uterus of an adult woman consists of an outer layer of connective tissue and smooth muscle known as the myometrium and an inner, softer, more vascular endometrium that is sloughed every twenty-eight days. Deeper than the endometrium is the uterine cavity, which is no larger than a slit in the nonpregnant female but is capable of expanding to accommodate a baby weighing seven or eight pounds or more.

Scientists are still making discoveries about the functions of the uterus independent of supporting a fetus. It is known to produce two vital groups of chemicals. The first of these are beta endorphins, the body's natural painkillers, which produce a mild euphoria and sense of well-being. The second group, the prostaglandins, serve a variety of functions. Because they cause contraction of smooth muscle, it is the prostaglandins that are to blame for menstrual cramping. They are also believed to be protective against heart disease because of their role in preventing blood clotting.

Branching out from the fundus, or top of the uterus, on either side are the fallopian tubes. Four inches long, they attach to the uterus via a nearly microscopic opening, and then end, just short of the ovaries, with finger-like projections called fimbriae. As mentioned earlier, the fallopian tube (also called the oviduct, or egg tube) is the vestibule between the ovary and uterus where sperm unites with egg. Fallopian tubes in the mature female have more glandular tissue than those in pubescent or prepubescent females. In addition, following puberty, fallopian tubes contain greater numbers of increasingly active cilia, which are constantly beating in the direction of the uterus. This obviously aids the ovum in its monthly journey.

Perhaps the most critical and complex of the female reproductive organs are the ovaries. Almond-shaped and weighing about a quarter of an ounce each, they rest in the pelvic cavity adjacent to the fallopian tubes. To review, the ovaries contain thousands of egg-bearing follicles—the sites of estrogen, progesterone, and androgen production. They synthesize these steroid hormones using cholesterol as a building block. It is therefore theorized that active ovarian function prevents buildup of cholesterol in the arteries of the body and thus protects women from cardiovascular disease until menopause.

In addition to progesterone, women synthesize three types of estrogens: estradiol, estrone, and estriol, as well as two male sex hormones, testosterone and dehydroepiendiosterone. (All of these chemicals are present in men as well, but obviously in differing proportions. It is believed that the sex drive in the female is related to her level of the male hormone, testosterone.) Estrogens, progesterone, and androgens are also made, to a lesser extent, within the adrenal glands, small organs attached to the kidneys. Some very recent studies seem to indicate that women continue to produce estrogens and androgens even after menopause, both in the adrenals and ovaries, and that they may play a role in regulating blood pressure in addition to their already established functions.

Aside from the reproductive organs, increased output of estrogen from the ovaries during puberty causes changes in the adolescent's overall physical appearance. Her skin is softer and her body more curvaceous from selective fat deposition. She experiences the characteristic adolescent growth spurt as well as a molding of her pelvis into the broad, oval structure necessary for childbirth. Throughout her premenopausal life, estrogen will also stimulate new bone growth, safeguarding her against the ravages of osteoporosis.

MENOPAUSE AND YOUR CHANGING PHYSIOLOGY

Medically defined, menopause is said to have occurred if a woman has had absolutely no monthly bleeding for a period of at least one year. For most of human existence, most women did not live long enough to experience menopause. They generally died from infectious diseases or childbirth years before any decline in ovarian function. Therefore, the collective experience of women facing the changes inherent in menopause is very recent history, and much of it is still misunderstood. In stark contrast to our great-grandmothers who lived a mere century ago, women in their menopausal years are not simply waiting out their final years. They are active in society and often engaged in first or second careers after having raised a family.

Menopause has three distinct stages. The first, premenopause, is a time of steady decline in ovarian function. In much the same way as they begin in the teenage years, the menstrual periods are irregular and sometimes occur without ovulation. Before the onset of menopause, a woman may experience heavier periods, lighter periods, and/or erratic changes in the pattern of her cycle. As mentioned before, once she has had no periods for one year, a woman is considered to have undergone menopause. This means that she has no active follicles remaining in her ovaries. She can no longer conceive or menstruate. However, her ovaries continue to synthesize hormones in small amounts, and this is key to the other roles they play in her body, mainly related to heart and bone health.

Most women experience menopause, the second stage, in their late forties or early fifties. Like menarche, the actual age varies between individual women and may similarly be related to such factors as race, heredity, nutrition, and general health.

The final stage is postmenopause, when ovarian mass decreases by 50 percent and ovarian hormone production wanes. A decline in estrogen production causes several distinct physiologic changes in women. The obvious one is absence of menstrual periods; two notable others are hot flashes and drying of the vaginal walls with a loss of their previous elasticity. While it is not completely understood, estrogen seems to stabilize the blood vessels, preventing them from enlarging and shrinking in an irregular manner. When estrogen is no longer readily available, blood vessels dilate and constrict unpredictably, causing the sometimes sudden and intense sweating and chills that women experience.

In addition, just as they had developed during puberty, the breasts, pelvic organs, and vaginal area now shrink as fat and glandular tissue thin out. Thinning vaginal tissue is more easily irritated. This may lead to painful intercourse or an inflammation of the vagina sometimes called atrophic vaginitis. Estrogen, protective of the heart and skeleton, is no longer present to counteract the effects of arteriosclerosis and weakened bones.

Finally, women may encounter a host of psychological symptoms ranging from moodiness and fatigue to depression. Researchers are at work studying how much of this is physiologic and how much is environmental or emotional, related to such life events as children leaving home, spouses dying, disease becoming more prevalent, and so forth.

WHAT A PELVIC EXAM CAN TELL YOU

Some women hesitate to come in for their annual pelvic examination because they find it physically or emotionally uncomfortable. However, understanding what takes place during that exam and why it is important may help to allay some of the discomfort. A pelvic exam is actually an excellent opportunity to have a discussion with your practitioner about how your body works.

The annual checkup is more than a Pap smear. First, the external genitalia are examined for any signs of infectious or cancerous lesions. Then, the speculum is inserted to separate the walls of the vagina, thus allowing your doctor to view the cervix. A normal, healthy cervix is pink and round, with a tiny opening in its center. It is that opening that expands to four inches during childbirth to allow the passage of the newborn baby from the uterus. The cervix should be free of discharge, growths, and erosion. (A fleshy protrusion on the cervix may be a small fibroid or polyp.)

After locating the cervix, your doctor uses a small wooden stick called a spatula to scrape off a sample of the superficial layer of cells from the surface. These, along with cells collected with a cotton swab from the cervical opening itself, are sent to the laboratory for examination. The Pap test (named for its inventor, Dr. George Papanicolaou) classifies these cells into various types, which will be described in Chapter 6. At this point, other specimens may be collected—for example, to check for any suspected infections.

The speculum is then removed, and the doctor performs a bimanual examination. This is so named because it requires the placement of both hands—one inside the vagina and one on the lower abdomen—so that the uterus and ovaries may be palpated between them. An experienced practitioner can discover, by feeling the contours of these internal organs, whether they are normal in size and shape. It is usually during this portion of the pelvic exam that fibroids are discovered. Indeed, they may merely be a coincidental finding in a woman who is having no problems with her menses but who, on exam, is found to have an enlarged and irregularly shaped uterus.

Last, but not least, is the rectal exam. Many patients would prefer to omit this portion of the examination because they find it distasteful or uncomfortable, but it is absolutely essential. Especially in a woman whose uterus is angled slightly backward, the rectal exam permits the doctor to explore the underside of the uterus and to check for ovarian tumors. In addition, endometriosis usually finds its way to the cul-de-sac overlying the rectum; a nodular or lumpy sensation to the uterosacral ligaments in that area is a telltale sign of endometriosis. During the rectal exam, a simple and quick test for rectal bleeding may be performed. This aids in the diagnosis of certain gastrointestinal conditions, including bowel cancer. It is important to emphasize here that unless you have had a rectal exam, you have not had a complete pelvic exam.

* * *

We have seen in this chapter that a woman's body is a dynamic, ever-changing system and that sometimes these changes, while normal, can pose problems. How these changes may best be dealt with will be discussed in Chapter 9. For now, we move on to the disease entities, signs and symptoms women may experience when something goes awry in this intricate system of anatomy and physiology.

Suggestion for Further Reading

The New Our Bodies, Ourselves by The Boston Women's Health Collective (Simon & Schuster, 1984).

PART TWO

PROBLEMS YOU MAY BE FACING—ABOUT THE ALTERNATIVE SOLUTIONS

Yesterday morning I arrived at the hospital to find that the woman whose hysterectomy I watched last week was going back to the operating room for the third time. Last week they took her back to remove a blood clot from the site of surgery, and yesterday they opened her and cleaned out all the clotted blood and pus, which should probably have been removed the first time they took her back.

I found myself staring at the tubes coming out of the woman's belly and vagina, wondering if the women would be so willing to have surgery if they knew what was being done to them. No one should be asleep for surgery.

—MICHELLE HARRISON, M.D., *A Woman in Residence*

3

FIBROID TUMORS
OF THE UTERUS

*Woman, in the interest of the race, is endowed with a set
of organs peculiar to herself whose complexity, delicacy,
sympathies, and force are among the marvels of creation.
If properly nurtured and cared for, they are a source of strength
and power to her. If neglected and mismanaged, they retaliate
upon their possessor with weakness and disease, as well of
mind as of body.*

—EDWARD H. CLARKE, M.D., 1873

*Marlene had only just passed her thirty-first birthday when she first faced
needing a hysterectomy. For several years her menstrual periods had become heavier and heavier to the point that she now needed to use two tampons and a pad simultaneously. She not only dreaded the embarrassment
of a public accident, but wondered if she was at risk for toxic shock syndrome. She felt literally robbed of one week every month when she would
be practically incapacitated. Marlene's gynecologist diagnosed multiple fibroids and recommended hysterectomy to put an end to her misery. But although she was still single, Marlene hoped to have children someday. She
began to explore the alternatives to hysterectomy.*

Fibroids are responsible for approximately 200,000 hysterectomies per
year. The most common "benign" disease entities of the female reproductive tract, fibroids are present in anywhere from 30 to 50 percent of all
women between ages forty and fifty, afflicting twice as many black women
as white women. Women who have never had children also seem to be at
greater risk of developing fibroids, although no one really knows why. It
has been noted that estrogen may somehow play a role in fibroid growth
and development, because they are never seen before puberty, and seem to
shrink after menopause. In addition, fibroids tend to worsen during pregnancy, when estrogen levels are high. Furthermore, in the early days of

higher-dose birth control pills, users seemed to be more predisposed to fibroids (again due to the influences of estrogen?).

WHAT ARE FIBROIDS?

The term *fibroid* refers to the fibrous-like tissue comprising a fibroid. However, fibroids are actually smooth muscle in origin. That's why the more precise but less commonly used medical term "leiomyoma" is actually more appropriate (*leio* means smooth; *my* means muscle; and *oma* means tumor or growth).

No one really understands why or how fibroids develop, but they are believed to start out as one tiny smooth-muscle cell that goes awry in the myometrium (middle layer of the uterus) due to a genetic mutation. From there, a myoma may remain within the myometrium or insinuate itself into the outer or innermost layers of the uterus. Fibroids within the central muscle layer of the uterus are called intramural or interstitial tumors. Those on the outside protruding into the abdominal cavity are subserous or serosal types, and ones that invade the endometrium are called submucous leiomyomas (see Figure 3.1).

Fibroids occasionally migrate out from the uterus and invade the cervix, surrounding ligaments, or, rarely, other abdominal organs containing smooth muscle. (Fibroids have even been found in the stomach and intestine.) Like all living tissue, they require oxygen and nutrients transported to them via the bloodstream. Fibroids that develop a blood supply outside of the uterus are termed parasitic fibroids. Ones that elongate and grow a stalk (only submucous and subserous types) are called pedunculated fibroids.

Fibroids can be singular, but they are more commonly multiple. Some are so tiny that they are visible only under a microscope; some are large enough to weigh thirty pounds. Furthermore, a woman's symptoms may have no direct bearing on the number or size of the tumors—she may have one the size of a full-term pregnancy that causes her little or no discomfort! When women do complain of problems, however, the size and location of the fibroid will have a great bearing on fibroid management. For example, if a fibroid is sitting on top or beneath what appears to be a normal uterus, it becomes relatively simple to save the uterus. But in some cases the cavity has been tremendously elongated and distorted—sometimes actually curving itself around a fibroid—and then it's a judgment call as to whether hysterectomy would be the prudent choice. A complex myomectomy operation (surgical removal of just the fibroid while leaving the uterus intact)

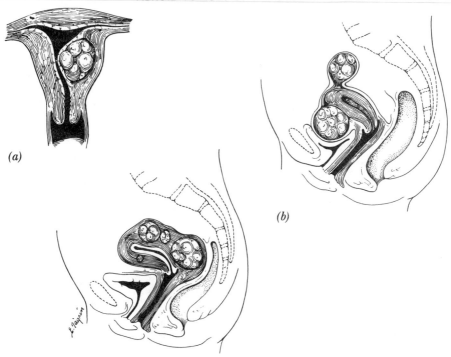

Figure 3.1 *Uterine fibroids*—Benign growths of muscle tissue named according to the location in the uterus: (a) submucous (inside the endometrium), (b) subserous (outside the uterine wall), and (c) intramural (within the uterine wall).

would certainly be worthwhile in a very young woman; the need to save her uterus should be measured against the complexity of the surgery. Some women have one large fibroid—a rather simple problem to correct. Others have as many as twenty or thirty tumors; in this case, removal of the uterus is often most prudent. For a woman in her forties who is not planning to have children, it becomes foolhardy to attempt to save a uterus that has the overwhelming potential and probability of continuing to bleed and cause her ongoing problems.

THE SYMPTOMS YOU MAY HAVE FROM FIBROIDS

Many fibroids are silent, meaning that they have no noticeable effect on your body. However, the following are the most common symptoms that you may experience as a result of your fibroids.

Symptoms of Fibroids

- Heavy menstrual periods (using more sanitary napkins or tampons than you normally use, or having to use two pads or tampons at once)
- Passage of blood clots
- Prolonged menstrual periods (lasting longer than previous menstrual periods; e.g., seven days instead of four)
- Painful menstrual periods. The pain may be dull and aching or sharp and intense; it may not respond to the usual drugs prescribed for menstrual cramps
- A sensation of heaviness in your lower abdomen, lower back, or legs
- Frequent or painful urination; the inability to control urinary flow
- Dizziness, weakness, pallor; fainting spells
- Problems conceiving or carrying a pregnancy to term

Bleeding

In general, heavier flow and perhaps more painful menstrual periods are the most common symptoms that women experience from fibroids. They may suffer from a gushing flow or the passage of blood clots, and may experience some of the signs of the anemia that heavy bleeding can cause, such as pallor, fatigue, or dizziness. However, fibroids can also cause an abnormal pattern of bleeding, such as staining between periods or bleeding after menopause. This is less common, and any woman having this kind of bleeding should not automatically attribute it to fibroids (even if she is known to have them). Other potentially more serious causes of abnormal bleeding have to be ruled out. (For the record, one-half of 1 percent of fibroids become malignant. From a practical perspective, in my twenty-five years of gynecological practice, I have seen only two patients whose fibroids were cancerous. A cancerous fibroid, or leiomyosarcoma, is suspected when a fibroid enlarges at an unusually rapid rate.)

Submucous fibroids may cause ulceration or distortion of the uterine lining surrounding them, which can then lead to abnormal bleeding. The severity of the bleeding associated with fibroids has a great deal to do with their location. For example, in contrast to subserous fibroids, which may cause few symptoms relative to their size, even a small intramural or submucous fibroid can cause hemorrhaging. This is because fibroids that extend through the thickness of the uterine wall and into the endometrium below have large blood vessels coursing through them. During menstruation, when the endometrium is sloughed, these vessels open up and literally pour out blood. Scores of patients suffering from these types of fibroids are afraid to wear light-colored clothing or even to go to work for fear of the opening of the floodgates during their periods. Ironically, as long as the blood supply to these fibroids remains so generous, these women may experience little or no dysmenorrhea (painful menstrual cramping).

Pain

About one-third of women with myomas (fibroids) have pelvic pain. As mentioned earlier, fibroids require blood to transport the nutrients necessary to maintain them. If the blood vessels are too few or too narrow, as when a large fibroid is anchored by a small stalk, there may be inadequate support to keep it viable and it may begin to degenerate. The death of the fibroid causes an inflammatory response as the body tries to rid itself of this dying tissue. Inflammation causes pain, usually in the form of cramping as the uterus contracts.

Depending on its location, a fibroid may cause different types of pain. A submucous fibroid, for example, may cause laborlike pains as the uterus tries to expel it through the cervix during menstruation. Pedunculated fibroids can become twisted on their stalks, causing sudden and intense pain as the blood supply is abruptly shut down. Intramural fibroids, like adenomyosis (a condition discussed in Chapter 4) may cause a generally tender, achy uterus. Finally, fibroids located on the outside of the uterus may impinge on other pelvic structures, causing so-called pressure symptoms.

Pressure Symptoms

Many women with fibroids suffer from a sensation of pressure in their back, legs, or lower abdominal region. For example, if a fibroid rests on vessels supplying blood to the legs, a woman may develop varicose veins and experience pain with prolonged standing. Fibroids located on the back of the uterus may cause backaches, rectal pressure, or constipation. Fibroids in front of the uterus may cause a woman to experience pain during intercourse or to urinate frequently. Bladder problems may abound with certain strategically located tumors—even causing conditions in which the woman cannot adequately urinate. Retention of urine predisposes a woman to infections because stagnant urine is a perfect medium for bacterial growth. Eventually, the urine within the bladder overflows uncontrollably, resulting in incontinence.

Pregnancy-Related Problems

Fibroids may be responsible for problems related to pregnancy literally from start to finish. There is significant controversy about whether infertility can result from the presence of a fibroid and if so, how. For example, if a fibroid is present within the uterine lining, it might cause interference with the implantation of the fertilized egg. Fibroids may also somehow interfere with sperm, cause distortions of the fallopian tubes, or change the position of the cervix and/or ovaries. Yet many women with fibroids conceive without difficulty. This leads one to believe that perhaps in women who don't conceive, another factor, such as blocked fallopian tubes or endometriosis, may be the actual cause.

The pregnant woman with fibroids requires expert obstetrical care and careful monitoring. Some experts maintain that when a fibroid is directly under the uterine cavity and lies on the same side as the pregnancy, the chance of miscarriage is very high. When the fibroid lies on the opposite side from the pregnancy, the chances of miscarriage are not high, except that the woman might have significant—even incapacitating—pain during the pregnancy. With small fibroids, the odds are on her side to have a safe, usually vaginal, delivery of a healthy baby. Larger fibroids may pose special challenges to the patient and her doctor. This is because uterine fibroids increase in size greatly during pregnancy (by approximately 32 percent) when estrogen levels are high, and this may place the woman with fibroids more at risk for miscarriage, premature birth, or postpartum hemorrhage.

Some women opt to have surgery performed prophylactically—in other words, to prevent problems with conception and pregnancy. Unfortunately, statistics reveal that only 50 percent of women who have myomectomies eventually conceive. Part of the problem is that in almost every woman who has abdominal surgery, tremendous adhesions (scar tissue) form after the surgery. If I perform a myomectomy in a patient who desires it for future pregnancy, I cover the scar with a Gore-Tex® patch to protect it against forming extensive adhesions. Ten days to two weeks later, I perform a follow-up laparoscopy to remove the patch and any adhesions that may have formed. If I wait a month or more, the adhesions will have become fixed, the procedure becomes very difficult and dangerous, and the chance of new adhesions forming is very high. Numerous studies have shown that higher pregnancy rates follow this procedure, and most reproductive specialists would agree. Unfortunately, this does mean additional minor surgery, but it is ambulatory and women can go home the same day.

TREATMENT OF FIBROIDS—
THE STANDARD RESPONSE

A "dusting and cleaning" is the patient's nickname for the ubiquitous D&C (dilation and curettage). Easily the most commonly performed gynecological procedure, literally millions are done every year. According to Dr. Michele Harrison, it is the "'bread and butter' of gynecologic surgery." After anesthetizing the patient, the doctor first inserts instruments to gradually widen the cervical opening and then uses other surgical tools, passed through this opening, to scrape away the endometrium. The gynecologist may also obtain tissue samples that will be sent to the laboratory in an effort to diagnose the cause of the bleeding.

The D&C has traditionally been a very popular procedure because it was believed to be both diagnostic and therapeutic for women with heavy menstrual periods or abnormal bleeding patterns. However, critics of the D&C, such as myself, believe that it's outdated and doesn't go far enough in helping women. To begin with, the traditional D&C is a blind procedure because the doctor doesn't directly view the uterine lining and thus must rely on what he or she feels with the curette to diagnose the presence of fibroids or other abnormal growths. Therefore, the gynecologist cannot be sure that he or she has eradicated the problem or sampled the key portion of the endometrium for lab analysis. Furthermore, the D&C hardly ever cures the bleeding. Specifically, my research as well as studies conducted by Dr. Frank Loffer have shown that at least one-third of pathology is missed during curettage. Dr. Loffer's work also demonstrated that a D&C provides only temporary relief of bleeding because it scrapes off only the superficial layer of the uterine lining. The foundation of the lining remains, allowing for a recurrence. As a result, many women need repeated D&Cs. The "standard response" after three unsuccessful D&Cs is hysterectomy!

Let's look at how modern diagnostic and treatment techniques have broadened the standard response to the management of fibroids.

THE MODERN APPROACH
TO DIAGNOSIS

In 1805 a German military physician of Italian descent named Philipp Bozzini became the first scientist to devise an instrument through which one could observe the hidden cavities of the human body. He called his invention the "Lichtleiter"; lighted by a candle, it was little more than a long, thin lantern made of tin and covered with leather. Although it received a brief flurry of publicity, including an endorsement from Archduke Karl, a member of the Austrian royal family, the Lichtleiter soon fell victim to politics and jealousies. Bozzini disappeared into obscurity, and it wasn't until 1869 that the idea of examining internal body cavities was once again raised—this time by a doctor named Pantaleoni. Pantaleoni first used his narrow tube and a kerosene lamp to examine the cause of heavy bleeding in an elderly woman. Over the next century, scientists and physicians continued to perfect various scopes to examine the genitourinary tract, adding more complex lenses, using cold light fiberoptics, and introducing fluids and suctioning devices into the uterus. Fluids and suctioning devices were used to minimize distortion from blood and debris, and to maximize visibility of the structures within the cavity. Today, the descendant of the Lichtleiter is called the hysteroscope (see Figure 3.2).

Hysteroscopy: The End to the Blind D&C

Hysteroscopy is a low-risk procedure during which the physician inserts a fiberoptic scope into the cervix—the lowermost portion of the uterus—in the presence of either a sugarlike fluid or carbon dioxide gas, which enlarges the uterine cavity, making it easier to examine. If you were to undergo this procedure, you would probably need only mild sedation and would feel little discomfort during the examination. No incision is made

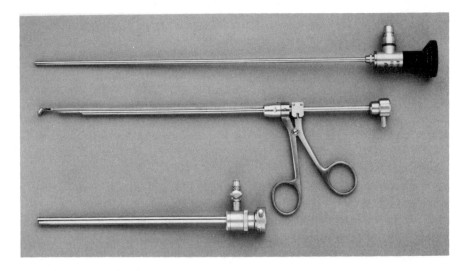

Figure 3.2 *A hysteroscope*—A fiberoptic scope inserted through the cervix to view the interior of the uterus.

and thus no scars are left. Hysteroscopy can be performed in a doctor's office or in the hospital. Afterward, you could go home and resume your normal activities in a few days. The side effects are generally very minor, and may include some mild cramping or light bleeding. Very rarely— about one in every ten thousand patients—a woman may have an allergic reaction to the sugarlike fluid used. I have begun to use an electrolyte solution called Ringer's solution because I believe it is the safest and most predictable in its properties.

The advantage of hysteroscopy over D&C, of course, is that the doctor is able to evaluate the entire lining of the uterus, and thus can usually determine the cause of the woman's symptoms. The gynecologist can not only detect polyps, fibroids, and suspicious tumors, but can sample the endometrium at the same time. Several studies now confirm what common sense seems to tell us: that hysteroscopy is more sensitive and more accurate than dilation and curettage. In a study published in the *American Journal of Obstetrics and Gynecology* in 1985, Drs. Goldrath and Sherman found that "large numbers" of polyps and fibroids were missed on blind D&C because "less than half of the uterine cavity had been curetted in sixty percent of patients and less than a fourth of the cavity in sixteen percent"!

In 1987 I published a retrospective study of nearly two hundred women evaluating the efficacy of D&C by hysteroscopy and found results similar to those of Goldrath and Sherman. In those cases, hysteroscopy was routinely performed prior to curettage. After identifying 185 patients with pathology such as polyps, I found that most patients still retained their polyps after curettage. Most required multiple attempts at removal. Only with hysteroscopy could I tell that the pathology had been completely removed. In addition, hysteroscopy spared patients the need to return for repeated curettages while continuing to suffer from their symptoms, because an examination of the entire uterus was able to be conducted at once.

Another advantage to this procedure is that instruments may be introduced via the hysteroscope to treat abnormal bleeding conditions, making operative hysteroscopy a simpler, safer, and more convenient alternative to hysterectomy for millions of women. Despite all of this, some physicians avoid hysteroscopy because of the difficulty they have viewing the uterine cavity when too much blood is present. Because of this problem, I have developed new techniques to make office hysteroscopy accurate and predictable even in the face of uterine bleeding. This work is described in a paper published in 1996 in the *Journal of the American Association of Gynecologic Laparoscopy.*

Abdominal and Transvaginal Ultrasound

Ultrasound (sonography) utilizes the emission of intermittent high-frequency sound waves that bounce off the structures within the pelvic cavity in certain patterns depending on the density of the structure. The patterns are then interpreted by a computer and conveyed on a television screen to depict the size, shape, and any irregularities of the uterus and ovaries. With respect to fibroids in particular, ultrasound can specify the number, size, shape, location, and consistency of myomas, but it cannot differentiate between a cancerous versus a noncancerous growth. Ultrasound is a very safe, noninvasive diagnostic test during which a physician or technician applies a conducting jelly to the abdomen and then passes a metal object called a transducer over it to record the sound waves. No dyes or X rays are involved. The test takes about thirty minutes to perform.

Traditionally, sonograms have been performed through the abdomen, allowing us to see an overview of the size of the uterus and the position of the myomas. The only discomfort to be anticipated is that a full bladder is required so that a clear view of the pelvic organs may be obtained. Abdominal ultrasound may result in a less-than-optimal picture in women who are substantially overweight or who have scar tissue or intestinal gas—all of these factors may obscure the picture. To overcome many of these obstacles, I use transvaginal ultrasound extensively in my practice.

During transvaginal ultrasound, a full bladder is unnecessary. A plastic probe covered with a lubricated latex sheath is inserted into the vagina, where it can then be positioned at different angles to directly view the uterus, ovaries, fallopian tubes, and the area behind the uterus known as the cul-de-sac.

Several studies support the notion that the transvaginal route permits a better quality image and provides more information to both doctor and patient about the status of her pelvic structures. For example, in one study published in 1988 in the journal *Radiology*, Dr. Ellen Mendelson and her colleagues compared transabdominal and transvaginal ultrasound in two hundred women. They discovered that transvaginal image quality was better overall in 79 to 87 percent of all scans. Specifically because the vaginal probe is closer to the organs being studied, one gets a clearer view of the uterus (including finer endometrial detail), the fallopian tubes (especially important when searching for an ectopic pregnancy), and the ovaries (except when they were in a high position). With respect to fibroids, transvaginal ultrasound allows us to see inside the uterine cavity and the lining of the uterus itself to determine if there are any fibroids present in those locations. The image quality of vaginal ultrasound is unaffected by abdominal scarring, obesity, intestinal gas, or a full or empty bladder. Because it is quicker and less uncomfortable for most patients, women tend to prefer this approach.

Transvaginal ultrasound will probably be the way of the future for most gynecologic ultrasound. The latest variant, fluid sonography, allows excellent visualization of the uterine cavity. It involves placing a thin, hollow tube called a catheter into the uterus and instilling saline solution into the cavity. A small balloonlike device is then inflated to prevent leakage of the fluid. The presence of this fluid clarifies the images seen via the endovaginal probe and allows us to see intrauterine tumors clearly.

Sometimes, a fibroid may be mistaken on ultrasound for other abnormalities. More expensive and more accurate imaging tests, including the CAT scan and the MRI, are occasionally performed to clarify the sonographic findings.

CATs and MRIs: The Alphabet Soup of Diagnostic Tests

CAT stands for Computerized Axial Tomography, a specialized form of X ray in which the organ being studied is X-rayed in a series of very thin sections or slices. The sections are then analyzed by a computer that assimilates them into a more three-dimensional and detailed view than is possible by conventional X ray.

MRI, or Magnetic Resonance Imaging, is the newest type of clinical imaging technique. Unlike the CAT scan, it does not use X rays; instead, it relies on a powerful magnet that exerts a force on the subatomic particles (protons) in the body tissue. Like the CAT scan, it utilizes a computer to analyze the patterns formed by the particles as they return to their normal state after being energized by the magnet. The detailed picture created by the computer is even more complete than those of ultrasound or CAT scanning.

TODAY'S TREATMENT OPTIONS

Today, a woman suffering from fibroids has available to her a variety of medical and surgical therapies to treat her condition—all of which thankfully fall short of hysterectomy. If you have fibroids, the therapy you select, in consultation with your gynecologist, is dependent on a variety of factors, including your age, symptoms, and childbearing plans. But before you select or agree to any type of therapy, you must get clear answers to the following questions.

Questions to Ask Your Doctor about Your Fibroids

- How did your doctor arrive at that diagnosis? (It should have been made via a pelvic examination with ultrasound confirmation and measurements, not merely based on listening to your symptoms.)
- How large are your fibroids, and are they likely to cause fertility problems? Women concerned with conceiving have a different outlook than women primarily concerned with avoiding surgery. (Remember, not all fibroids cause symptoms and some can be safely left alone.)
- What does your doctor suggest as the next course of therapy (if any is necessary)?

If your doctor suggests surgery, ask:

- What type of surgery does he/she have in mind and why?
- Does he/she perform hysteroscopy in lieu of traditional D&C? If not, find someone who does.

If your doctor suggests myomectomy, ask:

- Are the fibroids likely to recur before menopause?
- How will the myomectomy be performed—traditional open abdominal route, vaginal route, or laparoscopic procedure? (Opt for a surgeon who uses the most modern, least invasive procedure.)

If your doctor suggests hysterectomy, determine his/her reasons for choosing such a radical approach (especially if you have only mild or moderate disease, or other, less invasive procedures have not been tried). *Always seek a second opinion.*

- What are the consequences if you decide not to have the surgery?
- How long will you need to be in the hospital (if at all)?
- How long will you need to recover at home before you can resume your normal activities?
- What are the short- and long-term side effects of the procedure?
- What are the risks associated with this surgery?
- How many of these operations has your doctor performed?
- What is the fee for this procedure, and will your medical insurance cover it?
- Are there medical alternatives for shrinking the fibroids or ameliorating the symptoms?

If you are having abnormal bleeding and your doctor suggests a D&C, ask:

- How will this solve the fibroid problem?
- What will the next step be if the bleeding returns?

If your doctor suggests medical therapy, ask:

- How does this medication work?
- What are the potential side effects?
- Will this medication interact with other medications you may be taking?
- Is it contraindicated because you have other chronic medical problems?
- How effective is this medication?
- How long does the medication take to start working?
- Are the effects of the medication permanent?
- How long will you have to take the medication?
- Can the medication be self-administered?
- What are the costs?
- Will it influence your ability to become pregnant?
- What happens if you become pregnant while taking this medication?

Careful Observation

As already noted, chances are that more than half of women past age forty have a myoma, and many of them are unaware of it. Fibroids are coincidentally discovered on autopsy 50 percent of the time, suggesting that they are a silent presence more often than they are symptomatic. This is important to realize because it points to the fact that we do not have to intervene in every case where fibroids are discovered. Careful observation of the progress of that fibroid may be all that is necessary, particularly in a woman who is having no symptoms or who is nearing menopause.

When my patients fall into this category, I perform a baseline vaginal ultrasound, and then monitor them with pelvic exams every six to twelve months to follow their symptoms and any significant change in the growth of the fibroid. For example, if a woman has a fibroid that initially measured two centimeters (about three-quarters of an inch) and it doubles, it is still not bound to be a problem (providing she is having no symptoms). However, a four-centimeter myoma that doubles is significant, and a decision should be made about how to proceed. If the woman is young, a fibroid that size might interfere with a planned pregnancy, so treatment should be instituted to lessen the chance of complications. But if this woman is nearing menopause, she may elect to shrink the fibroid with medical therapy until the natural estrogen depletion associated with menopause takes over and causes the fibroid to recede permanently.

Medical Therapy—The GnRH or LHRH Agonists

In Chapter 2, where we discussed normal female physiology, you will recall mention of chemicals produced within the brain, notably in the hypothalamus and the pituitary, that influence the production of estrogen in the ovary throughout the menstrual cycle. Among the chemicals produced by the hypothalamus are gonadotrophin releasing hormone (GnRH) and luteinizing releasing hormone (LHRH). It is now possible for women suffering from fibroids (and a variety of other estrogen-dependent conditions) to take synthetic versions of these hormones to shrink their tumors.

Specifically, when a woman takes a GnRH agonist, usually via monthly, long-acting injections, she initially stimulates her pituitary gland to produce a follicle-stimulating hormone. This in turn causes the ovary to produce estrogen—as in the normal menstrual cycle. However, under the influence of these artificially introduced chemicals that constantly stimulate the body's sensitive feedback controls, the pituitary eventually (usually after a period of two weeks), becomes downregulated. This means that the bombardment of external chemicals mimicking GnRH has exhausted the pituitary's own gonadotrophins. Continued intake of the artificial hormone maintains that state. As a result, the ovary produces no estrogen and fibroids decrease to about half of their original size!

While a promising, nonsurgical approach to the treatment of fibroids, this therapy has some significant drawbacks. The first is that GnRH agonists to date have no convenient route of administration. They do not retain effectiveness when taken by mouth or as a vaginal suppository. They have to be injected monthly using what is known as a long-acting "depot"—a site underneath the skin where a long-acting version of the drug is implanted. They may also be administered as a daily nasal spray; however, a major drawback to its long-term use may be irritation of the nasal membranes.

Unfortunately, the GnRH agonists are not definitive therapy for leiomyomas for a variety of reasons. These medications are extremely expensive. Their long-term safety and efficacy have not been established; for instance, long-term estrogen suppression is known to cause osteoporosis.

But perhaps the greatest drawback to the GnRH treatment is its lack of permanence—as soon as treatment is stopped, most fibroids quickly grow back to their original size. One study followed women on GnRH agonists from the time they began therapy until from two to six months after they had discontinued the injections. While the fibroids had shrunk by anywhere from 62 to 100 percent of their original volume as long as the injections continued; once the medication stopped, 40 percent of these fibroids returned to their pretreatment size and in some cases actually exceeded it! (In this particular study, the statistics for shrinkage were higher than the generally accepted 40 to 60 percent decrease in size that one can find documented in most medical literature.)

At the present time, physicians are fearful of keeping women on these drugs for the long term because of the potentially harmful effects of years of estrogen suppression, in terms of heart and bone disease. Furthermore, the maximum effect is usually achieved in twelve weeks of therapy; beyond twelve weeks, fibroids don't get much smaller, but they may become softer.

Why pursue this form of therapy? First, women who are approaching menopause may use this therapy to avoid surgery altogether. Second, women who are unable to undergo surgery because of health complications might use the therapy until their complications can be overcome or stabilized. For example, during GnRH therapy, most women stop menstruating, thus allowing the body to recover from the severe anemia that heavy bleeding from fibroids has caused. Last, but not least, short-term GnRH therapy may be administered to all women facing fibroid surgery to lessen its complexity—the medication shrinks the fibroids significantly, lessens the amount of bleeding, and eases the removal of the tumors.

Surgical Treatment—Myomectomy Versus Hysterectomy

Myomectomy is a surgical procedure whereby the fibroid tumors are removed and the remainder of the uterus is preserved and reconstructed (see Figure 3.3). It has been performed for years when the patient desires children. However, because this surgery is more complex and time-consuming, traditional physicians recommend hysterectomy, sometimes with oophorectomy, to women in their forties as a more "appealing" and permanent solution to their fibroid problem. It is true that once the uterus is gone, the fibroids will have no opportunity to grow back and cause any troublesome pain and bleeding. It is also true that hysterectomy is technically less difficult than myomectomy (though not to the doctor who is accustomed to performing myomectomy).

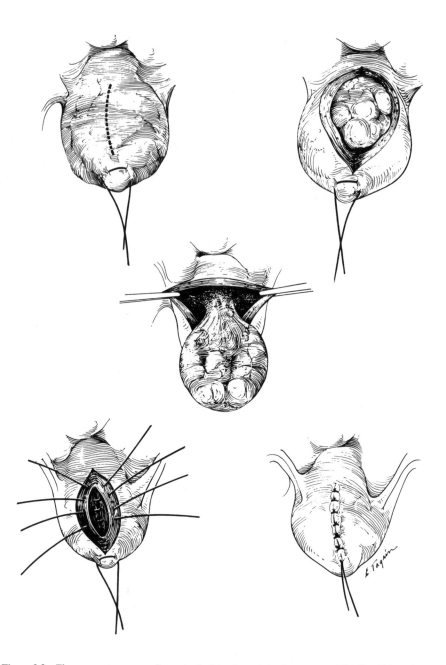

Figure 3.3 *The myomectomy procedure*—An incision is made in the uterus and the fibroid is excised, leaving the main body of the uterus intact.

Traditional physicians claim that myomectomy may cause greater blood loss and thus increase the need of a transfusion. Myomectomy results in a slightly higher death rate than does hysterectomy. And depending on the woman's age, the fibroids may recur. However, regardless of her child-bearing plans or potential, a woman may have physical and emotional reasons for wanting to preserve her uterus, and her feelings must be respected.

Claire, age 45, came to me complaining of extremely heavy periods. Though in agony, she was emphatic about keeping her uterus. After removing nine fibroids from her uterus, I was taken to task by one of my colleagues who could not begin to understand why I had not talked her into a more "sensible" hysterectomy. Yet, after her surgery, Claire was left with an essentially normal-sized uterus and was delighted when her next period was completely normal. Furthermore, she attained menopause without any recurrence of her symptoms.

Performed by a gynecologist experienced in uterine reconstructive surgery (as myomectomy is sometimes known), myomectomy is safe and may allow a woman to "buy time" so that she can complete her family or reach menopause—a time when her fibroids will recede and her symptoms lessen. In my opinion, there is certainly no age at which a woman "needs" to have a hysterectomy; only conditions that may warrant one. However, a woman must be well informed about her alternatives and her odds for success with myomectomy. Both are somewhat age-dependent. That is, if a thirty-year-old woman suffering severe pain and bleeding has a myomectomy, she may experience no further difficulties for ten years after the surgery. Now she's forty, is still menstruating, and has had ten symptom-free years with her uterus. However, for a forty-year-old woman who has a myomectomy, the chances are overwhelming that she will have no more problems, because menopause will intercede before significant regrowth can occur.

Although usually a myomectomy is an open abdominal procedure, depending on the size and location of the fibroids, it can now be accomplished by several different methods, including vaginally, laparoscopically, and via the hysteroscope.

VAGINAL MYOMECTOMY

Gynecologists can remove some intrauterine fibroids through the cervix and vagina, thus avoiding the risks and inconveniences of abdominal surgery. This technique is reserved especially for myomas with some degree of a pedicle (stalk).

Using local anesthesia to numb the cervix, the physician inserts several rods made of sterilized seaweed known as laminaria. Left in place overnight, the laminaria absorb fluid and swell, gently dilating the cervix. The next day, the laminaria are removed, and a specialized grasping forceps is introduced through the cervix. The forceps is attached to the fibroid and twisted, pulling the myoma loose, and removing it through the cervical os and out of the vagina. This procedure is best accomplished with relatively small, submucosal fibroids that have a stalk. Proper selection of patients minimizes the rare risk that the surgeon might damage the uterus or cause excessive bleeding.

Results of vaginal myomectomy compare favorably to the traditional abdominal approach. In one study published in *Obstetrics and Gynecology* (Ben-Baruch et al., 1988), bleeding was found to be much less and hospitalization stay shorter (an average of 2.4 days versus 7.8 days). In addition, in nearly 80 percent of patients followed for an average of over five years, no subsequent symptoms developed. In another investigation by Dr. Goldrath, vaginal removal of submucosal fibroids was successfully accomplished in eighty-three out of ninety-two women, with only six suffering complications (hemorrhage or uterine damage). The remaining nine women had fibroids that were too large to be removed in this manner. I am a disciple of Dr. Goldrath's technique and have found it to be extremely successful in well-selected patients.

LAPAROSCOPIC MYOMECTOMY

Laparoscopic myomectomy involves removal of fibroids through the laparoscope, a tube-shaped fiberoptic instrument that is introduced into the abdominal cavity via a small incision within the navel (see Figure 3.4). Like hysteroscopy, laparoscopy is ambulatory surgery with a minimal recovery period. It also requires the presence of a gas, carbon dioxide, which is instilled into the abdomen prior to the insertion of the laparoscope. This pushes other abdominal structures out of the viewing area so that the gynecologic organs may be clearly examined. Since laparoscopy is performed under general or regional anesthesia, the patient has no discomfort during the operation. Afterward, she may have tenderness at the site where the scope was inserted and painful cramping under her ribs or in her shoulder from gaseous irritation of nerve tissue. This abates in a few days once the carbon dioxide is absorbed by her body.

Risks are associated with laparoscopy. As with all surgery, there may be wound infections or anesthesia complications. In addition, rare accidental punctures of bowel or blood vessels may occur as the laparoscope is inserted.

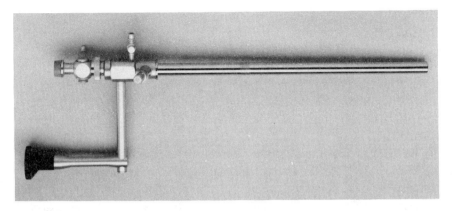

Figure 3.4 *A laparoscope*—A fiberoptic scope inserted via a minute incision in the abdomen and used to view the pelvic organs.

In reality, laparoscopic myomectomy is a difficult procedure to perform because of the complexities involved in suturing and in avoiding damage to the uterine cavity. This is especially important for women who want to preserve their childbearing capabilities. Criteria have been proposed for performing laparoscopic myomectomies. If the fibroid is small and superficial, it can readily be removed via the laparoscope. However, if the fibroid is deep and submucosal, it can impact on the uterine cavity; distortion in the cavity can cause some difficulty in suturing. Under these circumstances, I have serious reservations about doing a laparoscopic myomectomy because it might take four or more hours to complete, and that involves anesthesia risk and excessive blood loss. Fortunately, there are a host of other ways to deal with troublesome fibroids.

Myoma Coagulation, or Myolysis
This technique was first used in Europe in the late 1980s. I introduced it to the United States in 1990. It involves the use of a laser or special electrical needle to repeatedly pierce and destroy fibroids located within the uterus. Access to the fibroid is gained via the laparoscope. The term *laser* is an acronym for Light Amplification by Stimulated Emission of Radiation. This technique takes an intense and sharply focused beam of light and converts its energy from light to heat. This heat can then be used to cut, coagulate, or actually vaporize blood vessels or tissue. In the latter case, the moisture within the body tissue is converted to steam and literally dissipates into the air. Because the laser coagulates (seals off) blood vessels as they are cut, and because its tremendous heat significantly reduces bleeding, there is a decreased probability of transfusion. It is a much

quicker, less painful surgical procedure than either hysterectomy or myomectomy because it does not require a single incision. However, many hospitals cannot afford laser equipment, which costs well over $100,000. Because of this, I developed a special bipolar needle to accomplish what the laser does, and it has thus far proven to be equally effective in destroying the myoma tissue. This equipment is much more readily available in most operating rooms and is much less expensive to purchase, operate, and maintain.

By destroying the fibroid's protein structure and blood supply, whether via the Nd:YAG laser or bipolar needle, these tumors shrink substantially. In fact, because I pretreat my patients with GnRH agonists to decrease their fibroids' size preoperatively, I am able to reduce fibroid size by 75 to 90 percent. In a five- to six-year follow-up of women who have undergone my procedure, there were few complications and only a rare regrowth of fibroids necessitating hysterectomy. Furthermore, women can go home the day following the operation, which takes only about a half hour to perform, and they can be back to work in four or five days. However, because this procedure shrinks and denatures uterine tissue and thus weakens the muscle wall, it is not recommended for women trying to have children.

I have traveled extensively teaching and performing this new technique, and I have published numerous articles about it in the medical literature. The five-year results have been outstanding. Unfortunately, new ideas spread slowly, so we must persevere in disseminating this information to women who may be candidates—and to their doctors. You may need to become a sleuth to track down a doctor in your area who knows about and can perform this procedure. Try contracting the American Association of Gynecologic Laparoscopists (see Appendix) or your local hospital if it is a major teaching facility.

Cryomyolysis: A New Approach to Myoma Coagulation

Another new procedure not yet performed by many physicians in the United States is a variant of myoma coagulation called cryomyolysis. In this technique, an instrument called a cryoprobe is placed into the fibroid laparoscopically; then supercold liquid nitrogen (−160° centigrade) is used to generate a small ice ball that destroys the tissue by freezing. The Food and Drug Administration (FDA) has approved this technique, but as yet we have no long-term results.

Sometimes myoma coagulation is combined with another older technique called endometrial ablation. This is done when women have severe bleeding as a result of their fibroids.

ENDOMETRIAL ABLATION

You'll remember that in our discussion of fibroids earlier in the chapter, we said that the two most common symptoms are hemorrhaging and pain. Pain can be alleviated by shrinking the fibroid via a laser or bipolar needle inserted into the growth during a myoma coagulation. With laser or roller-bar electrode ablation (permanent destruction, or removal) of the endometrium (lining of the uterus), bleeding can be markedly lessened or completely stopped without ever having to remove the fibroids, let alone the uterus! If bleeding is the only problem, an ablation can be performed through the hysteroscope, avoiding any incision.

After giving a general or regional anesthetic, a saline solution is administered via the hysteroscope to enlarge the uterine cavity. Then, if laser ablation is desired, the laser specialist can employ the Nd:YAG beam to permanently destroy the offending tissue and blood vessels. The gynecologist has a clear view of the operative field via the hysteroscope, and is thus able to identify and sample any questionable areas.

More commonly today, an instrument (which is actually a modification of an instrument developed for urologists) called a *continuous flow resectoscope with a roller-bar electrode*, or *vaportrode*, is used to coagulate (denature the tissue) and thus destroy the endometrium (uterine lining). Using a loop electrode attachment, the surgeon can first shave down and sculpt out small fibroids so that the tissue is flush with the rest of the uterine lining before coagulating the uterine cavity.

While initially popular, the laser has now fallen out of favor because of its high cost and because its small field of focus makes the procedure much more time-consuming. By comparison, hysteroscopic resection, using instruments such as the resectoscope, cuts operative time to one-quarter of that previously required when using the laser to achieve comparable results.

Other methods of endometrial ablation include the hot water technique, the vestibulate technique, and the cryoprobe technique. The first two are relatively new ideas that are being tested, but as of this writing have not yet gained FDA approval. Both procedures have the advantage of being reasonably noninvasive and thus can be done in the doctor's office instead of the hospital. In the hot water technique, a special balloon is inserted into the uterine cavity and filled with boiling water, literally cooking the endometrium and thus destroying it. Likewise, the vestibulate procedure involves a balloon fitted with special electrodes that can also be utilized to ablate the uterine lining. The drawback to both of these procedures is that because they use a balloon, the uterus must be relatively small and regularly shaped—which is frequently not the case when fibroids are present. The cryoprobe (see the section on cryomyolysis) is being used in certain centers to perform endometrial ablations on women who are quite ill and cannot tolerate general anesthesia.

Ablation of the endometrium is a wonderful answer for many women with heavy bleeding because it destroys both the lining of the uterus and its roots but does not cause the woman to undergo a premature menopause with all its inherent symptoms and problems. A woman will simply be unable to respond to her hormonal function, and thus she won't bleed at all or her bleeding will be significantly reduced.

It must be emphasized that this procedure *permanently* destroys the endometrium and thus effectively sterilizes the woman. Therefore, it is not an option for women who still want to have children. In addition, endometrial ablation is thought not to be appropriate for women in whom suspicious tissue was found on initial sampling of their endometrium by diagnostic hysteroscopy. This is because there may be isolated remnants of endometrial tissue left or able to regenerate after the ablation, and so it is still possible to develop an endometrial cancer. Abnormal uterine bleeding (such as postmenopausal bleeding) is a symptom of endometrial cancer, but 60 percent of women who have had the procedure will never bleed again. Therefore, this important symptom of cancer would be eliminated, and neither the patient nor the gynecologist would want that. Think of the analogy of a patient who is developing abdominal pain on her right side. The last thing a doctor wants to do is give painkillers to mask her pain and hence possibly cause him or her to miss a rupturing appendix!

Again, it is important to emphasize that while endoscopic specialists are concerned about and recognize this potential problem, in reality there have been only two reported cases of uterine cancer after endometrial ablation in the fifteen years gynecologists have been performing the surgery. In one of the two cases, the woman already had precancerous changes prior to the ablation, which should have been picked up on endometrial biopsy—a diagnostic procedure that should always be done prior to proceeding with ablation. In fact, one might also theoretically argue (again, this has never been proven) that because women who have undergone ablations have less endometrium (the aim of the procedure is to destroy the entire endometrium, but areas regenerate in 40 to 50 percent of patients), they have less chance of developing endometrial cancer! Nevertheless, it is my opinion that a woman with endometrial cancer will still bleed, even after ablation, and that if yearly exams demonstrate that her uterine cavity has not inadvertently sealed off, thus blocking the exit of blood through the vagina, she will be aware of that very significant symptom. To assure that no cancer will be missed after an ablation, I routinely monitor my patients once a year with an ultrasound to check for any blood collection within the uterus. In addition, one month after an ablation, I perform an endosuction procedure whereby I place a suction catheter into the uterine cavity to remove any debris that may be left inside and to assure that the uterine and cervical canal is patent. I must reemphasize that in my experience, many women still menstruate after an ablation, but the bleeding is markedly reduced.

Endometrial ablation offers a safe, simple, long-term alternative to open abdominal surgery for women with submucosal or intrauterine fibroids. It results in the complete elimination of menstrual periods for at least half of all women, with the vast majority of the rest experiencing, if nothing else, normal, manageable monthly menstrual cycles until they reach menopause.

STRATEGIES FOR TREATING SUBMUCOSAL AND INTRAUTERINE FIBROIDS

Once a month I see a young woman with extremely heavy bleeding whose uterus is only marginally enlarged. She usually comes in with an ultrasound study in hand and a report saying "moderate-sized fibroid." Trying to diagnose the position of a myoma from a report is like an engraver trying to work blindfolded. I need to see the mass in relation to the uterus for maximum information.

When an endovaginal scan with fluid instillation is done, a solitary intrauterine tumor is often found. If this tumor has a stalk, it can be easily removed. Otherwise, a GnRH agonist is used to shrink the uterine wall around the tumor and so internalize the tumor. Then operative hysteroscopic techniques can be used to remove the tumor vaginally and restore the patient's fertility and normalize her menses. Treating these patients is extremely rewarding because often they have been offered only abdominal surgery—usually hysterectomy.

Tumors that are in the muscle wall underneath the uterine cavity causing heavy bleeding are the most difficult to treat. Again, we use a GnRH agonist to reduce the blood supply, and if fertility is desired, we must resort to abdominal surgery with a laparoscopic follow-up procedure. If the patient is past childbearing, then endometrial ablation is performed. Myoma coagulation is also added if the tumor is relatively large.

More superficial tumors are easily destroyed by the laparoscopic coagulation technique. Laparoscopic myomectomy is sometimes used but only in selected cases, as I have previously described. All of these techniques require a well-trained, highly skilled endoscopic surgeon. It's therefore a good idea to consult the American Association of Gynecologic Laparoscopy to find a certified endoscopic specialist in your area.

* * *

Fibroids are women's most common and troublesome gynecologic complaint. The pain and bleeding caused by fibroids lead millions of sufferers to undergo hysterectomy each year. We now have specialized diagnostic and treatment techniques that can help a woman to preserve her uterus into menopause, when the symptoms of fibroids naturally abate from the withdrawal of estrogen.

Even significantly sized myomas can be safely managed by observation, as long as the fibroids do not cause excessive bleeding and the patients do not wish to become pregnant. These women need only be carefully monitored with periodic pelvic exams and ultrasound. However, women whose myomas cause severe bleeding, pain, and a significantly enlarged, irregular uterus may require myolysis and/or endometrial ablation or myomectomy as a more permanent solution to the embarrassment, discomfort, and ane-

---

Choosing the Right Doctor

- You should feel comfortable with your doctor. Remember, you and your doctor are making crucial, sometimes lifelong, decisions. You should feel that you were not rushed, that you were treated as an individual, that the doctor listened to your questions and concerns, and that he/she addressed them to your satisfaction. Make sure you feel at ease with the doctor's office and staff.
- Always seek a second opinion for a serious problem or when surgery is suggested. A second opinion should come from an independent physician who has no relation to your doctor.
- Be wary of a doctor who paints too rosy a picture—one that seems unrealistic—who gives you absolute guarantees, who seems cavalier about surgery and easily dismisses your problem or the surgery as "no big deal."
- Don't rush into major surgery unless you are convinced (by more than one doctor) that it is truly an emergency. Try to explore all of the alternatives first, and attempt to preserve your uterus if you can.
- Select a doctor who is a member of the American Association of Gynecologic Laparoscopy (see Appendix).

mia associated with their monthly cycles. A cautionary note: If other conditions are present in addition to fibroids, myomectomy or ablation may not be the answer. (This is especially true if adenomyosis is the problem, as we shall see in Chapter 4.)

This simple explanation is not meant to substitute for the highly individualized consideration each woman's case must be given in terms of choosing the treatment plan that is right for her. For some women, hysterectomy is the correct course, or it's the one that they desire. Others demand the minimal intervention that will solve their problem. The number-one job of the gynecologist is to address the patient's needs and desires, and to put into perspective for her, within the context of those needs and desires, what her chance of success will be when availing herself of any particular plan of care. Today, when so many alternatives are available and so much is known about the consequences of hysterectomy, a gynecologist who just says, "You don't need your uterus; let's take it out," is making statements both uncaring and unwarranted.

4

ENDOMETRIOSIS AND ADENOMYOSIS

Endometriosis is without question one of the most puzzling conditions that affect women. More is being learned about it as time goes on, and this knowledge is dispelling some of the assumptions of the past that now have been disproven or are suspect. . . . Perhaps someday soon we will understand this perplexing disease and be able to end all the myths, pain, and frustrations that sometimes go with it!
>   —MARY LOU BALLWEG, cofounder, president,
>   and executive director
>   of the Endometriosis Association

Today, it is extremely rare that any woman should need a hysterectomy for endometriosis, no matter how severe the condition. But this was not always the case. Consider Carol's situation:

Carol's symptoms began when she was in high school. Three or four days out of every month she would be bedridden with severe menstrual cramps. She felt helpless and frustrated—always wondering why she had been singled out to endure this agony. When Carol's schoolwork began to suffer as a result of absenteeism, her mother took her to see a gynecologist. Carol's mother had endometriosis, and she began to suspect that she had passed on this dreaded condition to her daughter. The doctor confirmed that Carol indeed had endometriosis and began hormonal therapy immediately. Unfortunately, Carol did not respond well to the medication, and her disease continued to progress. Exploratory surgery at age twenty-five revealed extensive endometriosis, with invasion of most of her pelvic organs. A short time later, she underwent a total abdominal hysterectomy with bilateral oophorectomy. While this finally put an end to her pain, Carol, now forty-four, is still very bitter about the experience. "I was never able to have children, and as a result, I feel I am lacking an experience that is an essential part of being a woman."

As we shall see, pain and infertility are a large part of the misery that accompanies endometriosis. Fortunately, the latest scientific advances in medicine and surgery can help women to overcome this common, invasive disorder.

ENDOMETRIOSIS—STILL AN ENIGMA

Physicians and pathologists first described endometriosis over a hundred years ago, and the landmark papers still quoted today by many gynecologists were written in the 1920s by the eminent American gynecologist John Albert Sampson. Yet, many of the questions we have about endometriosis are as shrouded in mystery today as they were during the last century. For example, while we do have a working definition of endometriosis, we are still not completely sure what causes it, or how it spreads (to areas as remote as the brain). Nor do we understand why adenomyosis, which is basically internal endometriosis, behaves so differently within the uterus from the way it does at remote sites, or why it afflicts a totally different group of women (see page 94 for an explanation of adenomyosis). Simply defined, endometriosis is the presence of viable, proliferating endometrium outside its normal site, the lining of the uterus. Most commonly, the so-called glands and stroma that comprise the endometrium migrate to the ovaries and the fallopian tubes. The next most common sites (in descending order of incidence) are the external surface of the uterus, the uterosacral ligaments (elastic fibers that connect the lower portions of the uterus to the sacrum), the area between the vagina and the rectum (called the rectovaginal septum), the cul-de-sac (the area behind the uterus), and the cervix, vulva, and vagina. However, endometriosis does not always limit itself to the pelvic cavity. Implants have been found in both large and small intestine, the bladder, breasts, arms, legs, lungs, and even the brain! Just like the normal endometrium, these implants bleed cyclically every month. They have been responsible for such bizarre and frightening symptoms in their unwitting sufferers as coughing up blood during the menstrual cycle (when implants are located in the lung, for instance).

When this aberrant tissue has enlarged to a size sufficient to categorize it as a tumor, it is called an endometrioma; otherwise, the growths are simply known as implants. Because of its invasive nature and the bleeding it causes, endometrial tissue has frequently been mistaken for cancer. Although endometriosis may riddle the body with tumors, wreaking havoc on the various structures to which it spreads, endometriosis is neither cancerous nor precancerous. This is certainly reassuring, but it does not minimize the damage and discomfort endometriosis can cause.

The Fallacy of the "Career Woman's Disease"

Mary Lou Ballweg, an endometriosis sufferer herself, and one of the most prominent names in the field because she heads a large organization dedicated to education and support groups for this condition, points out that there were and still are a host of false assumptions about who gets endometriosis and why:

> One of these past assumptions was that nonwhite women did not generally get endometriosis.... Another myth about endometriosis was that very young women did not get it.... It was also believed in the past that endometriosis more often affected well-educated women.... Another assumption that has at times been made about endometriosis is that it is not a serious disease because it is not a killer like cancer.... However, anyone who has talked with many women with endometriosis about their actual experiences with the condition soon learns that while some women's lives are relatively unaffected by it, too many others have suffered severe pain and emotional stress, have been unable to work or carry on normal activities at times, and have experienced financial and relationship problems because of the disease.

Julia Older, author of *Endometriosis*, a well-known book aimed at women like herself who had to make the unwanted odyssey through this disease, explains:

> Endometriosis sufferers are defined with a plethora of observations about behavior, psychological makeup, and personality traits. The professionals making the observations ... see women in pain, women anxious to have families, women who have had miscarriages, women who must make decisions about hysterectomies.... Most of the ... statements from medical texts and interviews are buried in scientific language. They have an aura of authority and thus a ring of authenticity to them. Santa Claus is always round and jolly. Women with endometriosis are always trim and aggressive.

Even the late Dr. Robert Kistner, a pioneer in the treatment of endometriosis, was guilty of stereotyping women: "I've rarely seen a fat woman with endometriosis. It's that type of individual who simply has to clean out the ashtrays all the time." Kistner provides a classic textbook description of the patient with endometriosis in the 1986 edition of *Gynecology: Principles and Practices:* "The median age of patients at the time of diagnosis is approximately 30 years. It is likely that endometriosis is more common in upper-middle-class professional women. Delayed and infrequent pregnancies may account for this association." Many gynecologists paint a similar picture. Consider the experiences of Joanne, who fit the picture perfectly when she was diagnosed with endometriosis:

Joanne is a 35-year-old upper-echelon marketing executive who was recently married and is living in Manhattan. She suffered for several years with pain during menstruation and with intercourse. However, she managed to find expert medical care, and a combination of medication and laser surgery has reversed her disease to a large extent.

Yet Joanne is very distressed about what she perceives as the syndrome of "blaming the victim" that occurs with endometriosis: "The first gynecologist I saw told me that I had endometriosis, the 'career woman's disease.' He implied that I had developed it because I was pursuing a career instead of being home raising a family. This was before I had even met Rick, my husband. He made me feel guilty that I hadn't married young and become pregnant right away, as if this had even been an option for me."

Endometriosis is found in approximately 5 to 15 percent of all women age twenty-five to thirty-five who undergo exploratory surgery for other causes, and in 30 to 45 percent of infertile women undergoing laparoscopy as part of their diagnostic workup. (We will discuss laparoscopy in more detail later in this chapter.) However, the symptoms and pathology begin much earlier in life (usually in the teen years) for many women. The principal symptom, severe menstrual cramping, may be written off by parents and physicians as psychological, or as an adolescent attention-getting device. And it may be that the reason endometriosis is frequently diagnosed in upwardly mobile, well-educated career women is that they have the resources to seek sound medical care. Finally, much of the evidence about pregnancy ameliorating the disease is anecdotal. Many sufferers have had children, and may have found that the endometriosis further complicated both their disease and their pregnancy. Furthermore, the oft-quoted low pregnancy rates among endometriosis patients may be a consequence, not a cause, of the disease. In fact, endometriosis is found in women of all ages, races, socioeconomic groups, and occupations. It has been diagnosed in women who have had several children as well as in women who have never been pregnant.

Putting aside demographics, women with endometriosis may share some menstrual characteristics. A large study conducted by Daniel Cramer and his associates involving over four thousand women revealed that "women with short cycle lengths (less than or equal to twenty-seven days) and longer flow (greater than or equal to one week) had more than double the risk for endometriosis compared with women with longer cycle lengths and shorter duration of flow." These women also tended to have begun menstruating at a younger age, and to report greater menstrual pain. The latter finding may be one of the characteristics the authors admit may be a "consequence" rather than a "precursor" to the disease. In any case, it is still helpful in identifying high-risk patients. The authors conclude that the "risk for endometriosis may relate to menstrual factors that predispose to greater pelvic contamination with menstrual products and to constitutional factors that influence endogenous hormonal levels." Here, they are probably alluding to another interesting finding in their investigation—that long-term heavy smokers and strenuous exercisers are less likely to develop endometriosis. (This is just an epidemiologic fact. Obviously, I am not advocating smoking as prevention or therapy for endometriosis, but exercise can only help you!)

Cramer's findings that a longer, less painful cycle with less bleeding results in less endometriosis dovetails with a 1988 report in *Obstetrics and Gynecology* by Brian Kirshon and Alfred Poindexter that looks at the effects of various contraceptive methods on endometriosis. As one might expect, former users of intrauterine devices (IUDs) had a significantly higher rate of endometriosis than did women who took birth control pills. The IUD is known to cause longer, heavier, and more painful periods. It is also documented to cause an inflammatory reaction within the uterus. (This, in fact, may be one of its mechanisms of action in preventing pregnancy.) The birth control pill, however, thins out the endometrium, and thus periods tend to be short and scant. This relative presence or absence of heavy bleeding leads us to explore the first, and perhaps the most popular, theory about the true underlying cause of endometriosis.

Retrograde Menstruation

Normally, at the time of menstruation, the cervix relaxes and the uterus contracts to expel the endometrial lining that has built up during that particular cycle. Just the opposite scenario is believed to occur in women with endometriosis; in other words, the lower portion of the cervix goes into spasm, impeding the egress of blood from the vagina. Instead, the blood is forced upward through the uterus and out the oviducts. It eventually winds up in the pelvic cavity where fragments of endometrial tissue can deposit around the fallopian tubes and ovaries, or it can fall by gravity to the bottom of the pelvis and remain near the rectum or in the cul-de-sac. This so-called retrograde menstruation has been observed on numerous occasions when laparoscopies were performed on menstruating women. These en-

dometrial "seedlings" then adhere to their surrounding structures and be-
have just as they would within the uterus: bleeding every month during
menstruation. These bleeding adhesions can cause serious problems, as we
shall see in the section dealing with the symptoms of endometriosis. Like
the authors of the two scientific studies mentioned above—Cramer, Kirshon, and Poindexter—many physicians believe that the heavier the menstrual flow, the greater the opportunity for endometrial implants to develop.

The theory of retrograde menstruation still leaves us with some of the
enigmas of endometriosis. For example, why is retrograde menstruation
observed in many more women than actually develop the disease? And if
endometrium escapes into the pelvic cavity during retrograde menstruation,
how does this explain the "renegade" tissue that has been found in such
mysterious places as under the arm or within the spinal column? The next
theory has been proposed to explain this latter phenomenon.

Blood-Borne and Lymphatic Spread

The human body has two complex systems of transporting materials
throughout its structure. The first and more familiar is the blood circulation, which is primarily responsible for carrying vital oxygen to the tissues
that comprise our organ systems and for removing the waste products they
generate. The blood also contains antibodies and specialized blood cells
that gear up the immune response whenever the body is threatened by a
foreign invader, such as a virus, bacteria, or allergen.

Like the bloodstream, the lymphatic system is vital to the body's immunologic defenses. In addition, it comprises a network of vessels, channels, and organs that pepper the landscape of our bodies with the mission
of collecting excess fluid that has escaped from the cells, tissues, organs,
and blood vessels. It is possible that endometrial tissue infiltrates these two
circulatory systems and is thus carried to remote and improbable sites of
the body where it implants.

Hypotheses to explain endometriosis abound, and ultimately it may be
discovered that there are many causes. The following are a few of the other
theories that have been advanced.

Coelomic Metaplasia

The term metaplasia refers to the differentiation of cellular material. It has
been suggested that certain tissue may retain its ability to differentiate into
other tissue under certain circumstances.

A fetus starts as a small ball of somewhat indistinct cells, but develops
embryologically into the various complex organ systems of the newborn.

What if the cells of the peritoneum (the lining of the abdomen) retained their ability to transform in the presence of certain stimulants? Specifically, what if menstrual products (as from retrograde menstruation) and/or hormones (estrogen and progesterone) could trigger the development of endometrial tissue where it would not normally be present?

This is the crux of the metaplasia theory, first described at around the same time Dr. Sampson was proposing his notion of retrograde menstruation. One very intriguing aspect to this theory is that it alone accounts for the rare instances when endometriosis develops in the absence of menstruation. Approximately 5 percent of cases occur in postmenopausal women, usually when they have been taking estrogen supplements. Likewise, the literature cites very rare reports of endometriosis in women who have never menstruated, and in men receiving estrogen treatments for prostatic disease. The common denominator here is estrogen administered from an external source, which may be the trigger for the induction of metaplasia.

Genetic, Immunologic, and Iatrogenic Factors

Your genetic background and/or the skill of your physician could have an effect on your risk of developing endometriosis and on your ability to control the extent of the disease! In *Comprehensive Gynecology* (1987), Dr. William Droegemueller discusses work that revealed that endometriosis was found seven times more often in the close relatives (mothers or sisters) of patients with endometriosis than in the relatives of patients without endometriosis. In addition, women with a genetic predisposition to endometriosis are found to develop the disease earlier in life, and to a greater extent than do women without fellow sufferers within the family.

One or more immunologic defects may explain why some women are particularly prone to endometriosis. Women with endometriosis seem to produce high levels of antibodies against their own endometrial tissue—a factor that may somehow play a role in the development of the disease. Another factor may be an abnormality in the body's immune response that causes it to fail to destroy wayward endometrial tissue. Another theory has to do with the role of prostaglandins (chemical substances that aid in the immune response): An excess of prostaglandins in women with endometriosis may be responsible for both the implants themselves and the severe cramping sufferers are known to endure.

Finally, endometriosis may be spread during the course of abdominal surgery, cesarean section, or laparoscopy. Implants have commonly been found at the sites of surgical scars and adhesions. However, as we shall see, improved operative techniques—including laser surgery—markedly reduce the incidence of physician-induced, or iatrogenic, endometriosis.

THE HALLMARKS OF ENDOMETRIOSIS

The following story tells of some of the common symptoms suffered by women with endometriosis, including pain, heavy periods, and sometimes problems conceiving.

"I couldn't concentrate on anything some days, the pain was so bad," confides Rochelle, a graduate student in clinical psychology. "I couldn't study or do my research. When I was interviewing clients, my mind was not focused on their problems. I'm the kind of person who's always on the move, involved with one project or another; yet, when I had my period, my husband would come home and find me lying in bed waiting for the latest round of painkillers to take effect.

"I suspected that I might have endometriosis. We read that pregnancy might put this into remission, so we began trying to have a baby. Months passed. The harder we tried, the greater the tension between us. For one thing, it was painful for me to have intercourse in certain positions. We went to see my gynecologist, who wanted to rule out other potential problems. All of the charting of my menstrual cycles and the battery of medical tests made sex more like a chore than a pleasure. Trying to conceive became a competition. It was us against this biological foe, endometriosis."

Pain

Pain is almost always associated with endometriosis. This pain commonly takes one or both of these forms: dysmenorrhea (painful menses) and dyspareunia (pain during intercourse). Throughout this chapter we have been discussing the enigmas associated with endometriosis, and here is yet another. Drs. Kistner, Droegemueller, and others have documented on numerous occasions that the more extensive the disease, the less severe are the symptoms and vice versa. I have personally seen a pelvis containing large or extensive implants that do not cause the woman any discomfort, whereas I've seen other women with only mild disease who are in excruciating pain. Of course, this is not always the case, and the extent of pain is not a reliable measure of the degree of endometriosis.

In addition to pelvic pain, women with implants located in sites outside of the pelvis will experience symptoms related to the organ that has been affected. For instance, implants located within or near the gastrointestinal tract may cause backache, abdominal tenderness, constipation, and pain and bleeding with bowel movements. Urinary tract disease may be associated with pain or pressure over the bladder and discomfort or bleeding with urination. The rare woman unfortunate enough to have endometriosis

within the chest may cough up blood or experience chest pain and short-
ness of breath.

The pain characteristic of endometriosis is cyclic. It is caused by the
swelling and discharge of endometrial glands into the surrounding structures. Both the swelling and the discharge cause a local inflammatory response mediated by prostaglandins. Unlike primary dysmenorrhea, which
is pain during menstruation without any obvious underlying pathology, the
secondary dysmenorrhea of endometriosis usually starts a few days before
actual menstruation and lasts longer into the cycle.

Dyspareunia, another characteristic of endometriosis, probably arises
both from direct pressure on endometrial implants that are low in the pelvis
and from the inability of the pelvic organs to move freely during intercourse. Often the endometriosis creates adhesive bands of tissue that bind
structures; when these adhesions impede the ovaries and fallopian tubes,
fertility is generally affected.

Infertility

Simply defined, infertility is the inability to conceive after one year of unprotected intercourse. Entire volumes have been written about the role of
endometriosis in infertility because it has been estimated that anywhere
from one-third to one-half of sterile women have endometriosis. In addition, these women have three times the risk of having a miscarriage if they
do succeed in becoming pregnant.

As we mentioned, endometriosis can cause the oviduct to lose its mo-
bility. Once it is unable to wrap itself around the egg and suction it into
its innermost portions, conception is unlikely to occur. Ectopic pregnancy
(implantation of the ovum within the fallopian tube) may also result because of this blockage that prevents the ovum from reaching its destination
within the uterus.

Aside from those severe cases where laparoscopy reveals the presence
of obvious endometriosis within the ovary or obstructing the fallopian tube,
the relationship of endometriosis to infertility is again a mystery. Some of the
theories that have been proposed—but never proven—blame hormonal imbalances, immunologic defects, and excess production of prostaglandins. And
of course, dyspareunia decreases the opportunity for conception to occur.

Bleeding

Although internal bleeding is the principal cause of the scarring and pain
associated with endometriosis, actual abnormal menstrual bleeding is present only in about 15 to 20 percent of sufferers. This is in stark contrast to

fibroids, where bleeding seems to be the major symptom that motivates women to seek treatment. If abnormal bleeding does occur with endometriosis, it is most common as spotting just prior to the onset of menses or as heavier flow during the menses.

DIAGNOSIS AND TREATMENT: THE STANDARD RESPONSE

We've talked about the symptoms, principally pelvic pain and infertility, that raise the specter of endometriosis for patients and their physicians. Once suspected, this diagnosis can be made on pelvic or rectal examination if the disease has progressed sufficiently. Tumors or nodules may be palpable on a bimanual examination of the ovaries or on a rectal exam of the uterosacral ligaments and rectovaginal septum. The ovaries may appear to be enlarged, and the affected areas may be tender to manipulation, especially when the examination is conducted during menstruation. Sometimes more sophisticated methods are needed to confirm a case where the signs and symptoms are not straightforward. In this instance, ultrasound and a diagnostic laparoscopy will almost always be undertaken.

Diagnostic Laparoscopy

Laparoscopy, as explained in Chapter 3, is a procedure that allows the surgeon to directly view your uterus, ovaries, and fallopian tubes without major abdominal surgery. Endometriosis may affect any or all of these structures, as well as various other internal organs, such as the intestines, ureters, or bladder. In mild disease, endometriosis may appear to be tiny purple or red ("blueberry" or "raspberry") spots. These spots may also be said to resemble powder burns. (See Figure 4.1.) Large endometriomas within the ovary are often called chocolate cysts because of the characteristic brownish appearance of the old blood that has accumulated within the tumor. (See Figure 4.2.) Recent investigations have shown that many nonpigmented lesions in the pelvis—previously overlooked—are indeed areas of endometriosis as well! The standard response on discovering endometriosis at laparoscopy would be to pursue hormonal therapy and possibly open abdominal surgery. However, as we shall see later in this chapter, through the combination of the laser, electrocautery, and/or newly developed surgical tools used via the laparoscope, women can now obtain immediate treatment in one simple procedure. First, let us explore the various treatment options offered by physicians following the standard response.

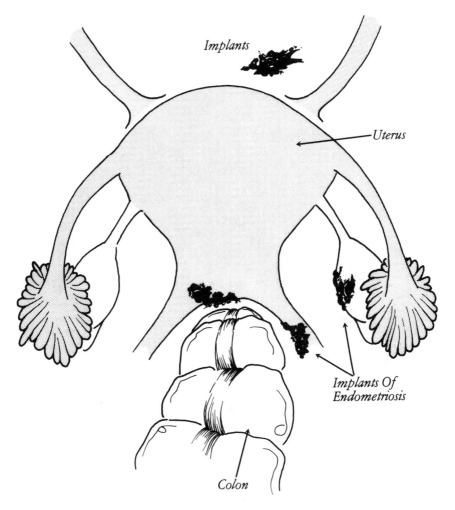

Figure 4.1 *Mild endometriosis*—Implants are small, flat patches of endometrial tissue growing outside of their normal location.

Prevention As Treatment

In *Gynecology: Principles and Practices*, Dr. Kistner very matter-of-factly states, "Early and frequent pregnancies appear to effectively decrease the frequency of endometriosis. . . ." Not only have we seen that this is a subject of controversy at the present time, but Kistner goes on to admit that "this therapeutic strategy is incompatible with the life plans of most patients." Therefore, setting aside pregnancy as an unproven and inconvenient treatment modality, we move on to the next best thing—pseudopregnancy.

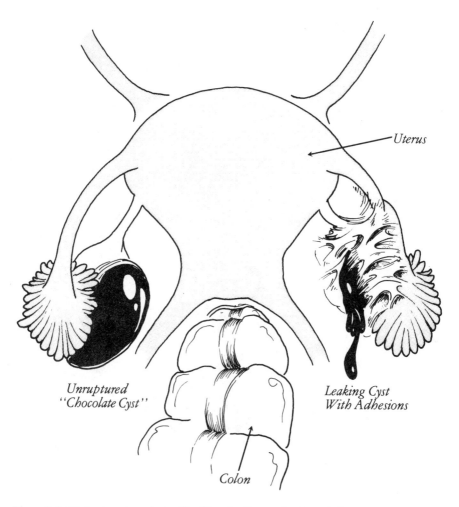

Figure 4.2 *Moderate endometriosis*—The "chocolate" cysts of endometriosis may be smaller than a pea or larger than a grapefruit.

Birth Control Pills and Pseudopregnancy

The use of oral contraceptive agents (birth control pills) to reduce the severity of endometriosis was first introduced over thirty years ago. They work both as a means of birth control and, in endometriosis, by fooling a nonpregnant body into functioning as if it were pregnant. In other words, the constant presence of estrogen and progesterone from the pill disrupts the intricate hypothalamic-pituitary-ovarian axis preventing ovulation. Without ovulation, the lining of the uterus doesn't build up and shed. There is no menstruation and hence no activity by the ectopic endometrium. The accumulation of tissue, pain, swelling, and bleeding that regularly occur with endometriosis are averted. This is accomplished by not cycling the estrogen and progesterone. In other words, normally when women are on oral contraceptives, the pills are cycled so that there is one week when the hormones are withheld and withdrawal bleeding occurs. In women with endometriosis, bleeding should be avoided entirely. To maintain this effect, a woman typically takes daily doses of estrogen and progesterone, and adds more pills whenever any breakthrough bleeding occurs. High doses of estrogen and progesterone initially cause the lining to swell, but after a few months the opposite reaction occurs: The lining atrophies and endometriosis recedes.

Twenty years ago, the high doses of estrogen and progesterone used to eliminate bleeding entirely could cause significant side effects, including very rare but serious ones such as the formation of blood clots in the brain, heart, or lung resulting in a stroke, heart attack, or pulmonary embolism. Less serious but still unpleasant side effects such as weight gain, headaches, and stomach upset combined with only moderate efficacy caused many women to abandon this regimen.

Today, low-dose oral contraceptive pills can be safely prescribed for continuous use (cycling them with three weeks on and one week off is no longer necessary)—a regimen that causes atrophy or thinning of the endometrium. The paradox is that oral contraceptives initially cause a swelling of the uterine lining, but over time the tissues become thinner and thinner. Less lining means less bleeding!

Because of problems with the high-dose pills of the 1970s, and the need for a newer, better treatment, the drug Danazol was developed and approved by the FDA in 1975.

Danazol and Pseudomenopause

Menopause, the total cessation of menstruation, has been observed to be a definitive therapy for endometriosis. Working with the model of menopause, researchers developed Danazol, which reduces estrogen levels quite low and induces a simulated state of menopause known as pseudomenopause.

Danazol is a derivative of the male hormone testosterone. As we mentioned in Chapter 3, one of its drawbacks concerns its masculinizing side effects. It may also cause breakthrough bleeding (vaginal bleeding at other times of the month besides menstruation), headaches, oily skin, mood swings, or gastrointestinal problems such as bloating. Danazol is also expensive. Danazol's major advantage is that like oral contraceptives, it allows for the control of endometriosis without surgery.

Danazol binds to the body's progesterone and androgen receptor sites and thus increases the amount of freely circulating testosterone present in a woman's system. Via another mechanism, Danazol increases the metabolism of estrogen and progesterone—that is, they are broken down faster in the body and thus are less available to carry out their respective functions. Danazol has also been observed to decrease levels of gonadotropin-releasing hormone as well as ovarian hormone production. The end result is that ovulation and menstruation cease. The lining of the uterus and all of its associated ectopic implants atrophy. Again, as with the Pill, pain from swelling and bleeding temporarily or permanently stop.

Danazol is the only drug that has a beneficial effect on the antigen-antibody reaction that occurs in the peritoneal fluid (fluid in the abdominal cavity) of sufferers. By decreasing the antibodies present, Danazol decreases any destructive effect these antibodies exert on sperm, thus theoretically enhancing a woman's fertility. In actuality, reducing antibody levels does not improve fertility, and women with endometriosis who take Danazol do not have a higher pregnancy rate than nonusers. However, if theories that endometriosis is an autoimmune disease are correct, Danazol offers women the only treatment that alters the immune response. It is also unique in its approach to the disease in that it reduces the inflammatory response of pelvic endometrial cells.

Treatment is generally continued with Danazol for six months to a year, depending on a woman's response, her experience with side effects, other medical conditions that may be present, and her desire to become pregnant. Danazol is very teratogenic (causing developmental malformation or monstrosities); therefore, it is imperative that women use a barrier contraceptive and avoid pregnancy at all costs while on this therapy. While Danazol does reduce implants and pain, it has not been shown to be effective in reducing infertility. In addition, it is not a permanent solution for many women. Unfortunately, recurrences can occur within one year of discontinuing therapy.

Combination Therapy

Sometimes Danazol therapy must be discontinued because the so-called therapeutic doses of 800 milligrams per day that have traditionally been given to women cause very significant side effects. Recent reports in the literature cite patients who have been able to take much lower doses (50 to 100 milligrams per day) to successfully control symptoms of endometriosis. I have begun prescribing this low-dose Danazol regimen along with Depo-Provera, a long-acting injectable progesterone. The combination causes a synergistic effect: Women do not bleed and their symptoms seem to regress. While there may be some bloating, the masculinizing side effects (such as the hot flashes) seem to be tempered by the use of Depo-Provera, which is a female hormone. I must make it clear that this is my own empirical technique—there have been no published studies on its effectiveness.

The "Definitive Therapy"

Dr. Kistner states: "For the patient older than 40 years with symptomatic endometriosis who has completed her family, the definitive therapy is total abdominal hysterectomy and bilateral oophorectomy." Likewise, "for the majority of patients with endometriosis involving organs outside the pelvis, total abdominal hysterectomy and bilateral oophorectomy are necessary." This is certainly "definitive therapy." In particular, removal of the ovaries precludes the proliferation of any existing or future endometrial implants. However, just as amputation of a leg will "cure" a severe infection and deformity that result from a motor vehicle accident, so may reconstructive surgery and intravenous antibiotics—obviously the more desirable choice.

Dr. Kistner was a highly respected pioneer in the field of endometriosis. He had impeccable credentials, and he set an example for every local U.S. practitioner wanting to know the proper management of this condition. Yet his statement concerning hysterectomy as definitive therapy represents the epitome of the outdated and rigid attitudes and thought processes of American gynecologists. Yes, it is true that hysterectomy with removal of ovaries will solve endometriosis, but unfortunately it also castrates the patient. If we castrate a woman in her thirties, she has to deal with the complications of that castration—estrogen deprivation. Then we have to replace the estrogen and progesterone in her system, which can reactivate the endometriosis. So it's a catch-22. Hysterectomy and bilateral oophorectomy in a premenopausal woman really do not solve the problems—because you end up creating other problems.

In defense of Dr. Kistner, when he first espoused this philosophy, adequate alternatives were not available and hence it was an appropriate therapeutic modality. The problem Dr. Kistner faced during his era was a lack of options. Operative laparoscopy was in its infancy, GnRH agonists were not available, nor were low-dose oral contraceptives for continuous therapy. However, we've come a long way in twenty years! Times have changed, and physicians should no longer take the easy way out for their patients. Every woman who so desires has the right to have her uterus preserved, given all the options presently available.

You are probably reading this book because you wish to avoid hysterectomy if at all possible. And as we shall see, today's repertoire of medical and surgical techniques provides viable alternatives for many women. Despite this, according to a large-scale government study, endometriosis was the only diagnosis for which hysterectomy increased between 1965 and 1984. It not only increased—it skyrocketed by 176 percent! This is because the standard response for physicians has been major abdominal surgery either after a failed trial of hormonal therapy or in combination with hormonal therapy. Within their protocol, the abdomen is opened and explored, and any evident endometriosis is excised. If symptoms recur, the next step after laparotomy is extirpation of all the pelvic organs. As Dr. Kistner further advises, "Large bilateral ovarian endometrial cysts with extensive peritoneal endometriosis and numerous pelvic adhesions or marked invasion of the rectosigmoid and rectovaginal space constitute the most urgent indications for radical removal of all the pelvic organs, regardless of the age of the patient." (See Figure 4.3.)

My approach to the treatment of endometriosis incorporates some of the methods employed in the standard response and expands on them. However, it deviates greatly in philosophy in that I believe that it is a rare woman who will wind up needing the so-called definitive treatment of hysterectomy. Today's treatment options are more extensive than ever, and they offer much hope to the woman experiencing the agonizing pain and infertility associated with this disease.

THE MODERN APPROACH
TO DIAGNOSIS AND TREATMENT

Treatment of endometriosis varies depending on the age of the woman and the extent of her disease. In an attempt to clarify the latter, several classification systems have been developed that divide endometriosis into stages. They all attempt to describe the extent of the disease from mild to severe by discussing the relative presence or absence of endometriomas, adhesions, and/or the involvement of organs outside the pelvic cavity. (See Figures 4.1, 4.2, and 4.3 and Table 4.1.)

Classifying the Disease

The American Society for Reproductive Medicine (formerly known as the American Fertility Society) has developed a widely used system of classification of endometriosis. (See Figure 4.4 and Table 4.1.) Points are assigned depending on laparoscopic findings. This system is an excellent

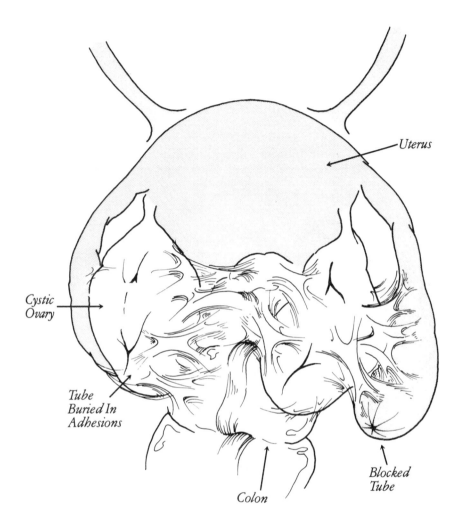

Uterus

Cystic Ovary

Tube Buried In Adhesions

Colon

Blocked Tube

Figure 4.3 *Severe endometriosis*—In some cases, bands of fibrous scar tissues (adhesions) bind the pelvic organs together.

method of scientifically quantifying endometriosis, but it unfortunately fails to capture the qualitative aspects of this disease. And it is the quality of a woman's life, the character of her pain and symptoms, on which we must base therapy in the everyday practice of medicine.

As with the standard response, pelvic examination, ultrasound, and laparoscopy are key components to the diagnosis of endometriosis. (Staging is based on laparoscopic findings alone.) In addition, MRI (see Chapter 3) is proving helpful since it can scan the blood-filled cysts and fiberoptic tissue that ultrasound and CAT scans lack the specificity to identify.

AMERICAN SOCIETY FOR REPRODUCTIVE MEDICINE
REVISED CLASSIFICATION OF ENDOMETRIOSIS

Patient's Name _____ Date_____

Stage I　(Minimal)　- 1-5
Stage II　(Mild)　　- 6-15
Stage III (Moderate) - 16-40
Stage IV (Severe)　- >40
Total_____

Laparoscopy_____ Laparotomy_____ Photography_____
Recommended Treatment_____
_____
Prognosis_____

PERITONEUM	ENDOMETRIOSIS	<1cm	1-3cm	>3cm
	Superficial	1	2	4
	Deep	2	4	6
OVARY	R　Superficial	1	2	4
	Deep	4	16	20
	L　Superficial	1	2	4
	Deep	4	16	20

	POSTERIOR CULDESAC OBLITERATION	Partial		Complete	
		4		40	

	ADHESIONS	<1/3 Enclosure	1/3-2/3 Enclosure	>2/3 Enclosure
OVARY	R　Filmy	1	2	4
	Dense	4	8	16
	L　Filmy	1	2	4
	Dense	4	8	16
TUBE	R　Filmy	1	2	4
	Dense	4*	8*	16
	L　Filmy	1	2	4
	Dense	4*	8*	16

*If the fimbriated end of the fallopian tube is completely enclosed, change the point assignment to 16.

Additional Endometriosis: _____

Associated Pathology: _____

To Be Used with Normal
Tubes and Ovaries

L　　　　　　　　　　　　　　R

To Be Used with Abnormal
Tubes and/or Ovaries

L　　　　　　　　　　　　　　R

For additional supply write to: American Society for Reproductive Medicine, 1209 Montgomery Highway, Birmingham, Alabama 35216-2809

EXAMPLES & GUIDELINES

STAGE I (MINIMAL)   STAGE II (MILD)   STAGE III (MODERATE)

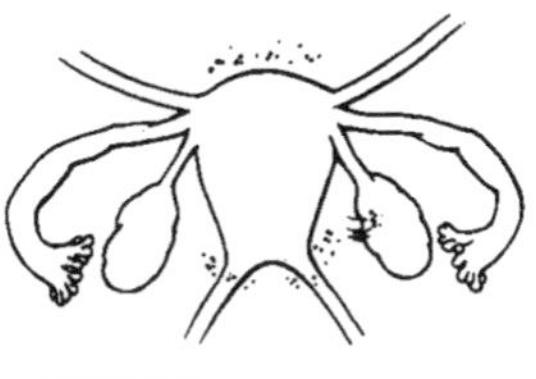

PERITONEUM			
Superficial Endo	–	1-3cm	· 2
R. OVARY			
Superficial Endo	–	‹ 1cm	· 1
Filmy Adhesions	–	‹ 1/3	· 1
	TOTAL POINTS		4

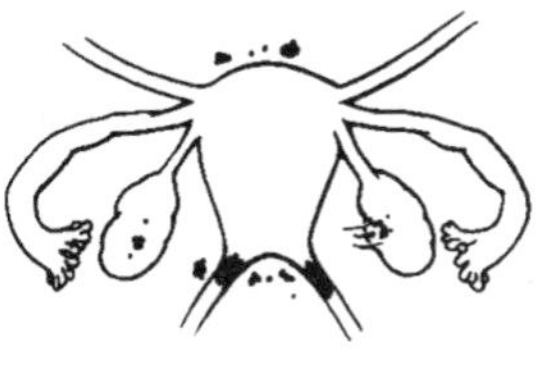

PERITONEUM			
Deep Endo	–	› 3cm	· 6
R. OVARY			
Superficial Endo	–	‹ 1cm	· 1
Filmy Adhesions	–	‹ 1/3	· 1
L. OVARY			
Superficial Endo	–	‹ 1cm	· 1
	TOTAL POINTS		9

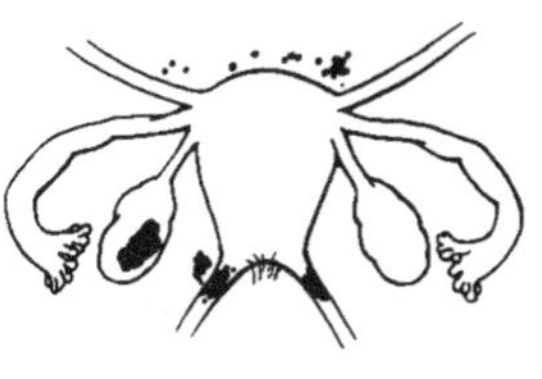

PERITONEUM			
Deep Endo	–	› 3cm	· 6
CULDESAC			
Partial Obliteration			· 4
L. OVARY			
Deep Endo	–	1-3cm	· 16
	TOTAL POINTS		26

STAGE III (MODERATE)   STAGE IV (SEVERE)   STAGE IV (SEVERE)

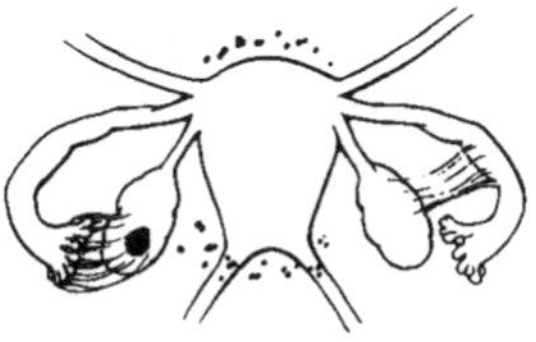

PERITONEUM			
Superficial Endo	–	› 3cm	-4
R. TUBE			
Filmy Adhesions	–	‹ 1/3	· 1
R. OVARY			
Filmy Adhesions	–	‹ 1/3	· 1
L. TUBE			
Dense Adhesions	–	‹ 1/3	· 16*
L. OVARY			
Deep Endo	–	‹ 1 cm	-4
Dense Adhesions	–	‹ 1/3	-4
	TOTAL POINTS		30

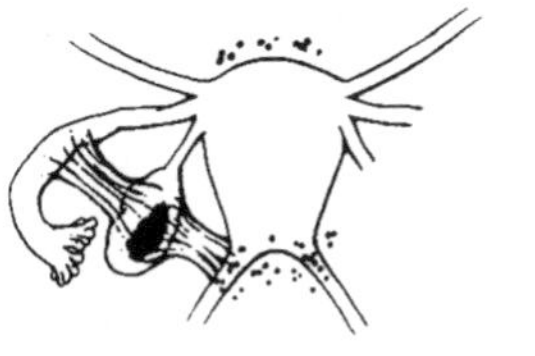

PERITONEUM			
Superficial Endo	–	› 3cm	-4
L. OVARY			
Deep Endo	–	1-3cm	· 32**
Dense Adhesions	–	‹ 1/3	· 8**
L. TUBE			
Dense Adhesions	–	‹ 1/3	-8**
	TOTAL POINTS		52

*Point assignment changed to 16
**Point assignment doubled

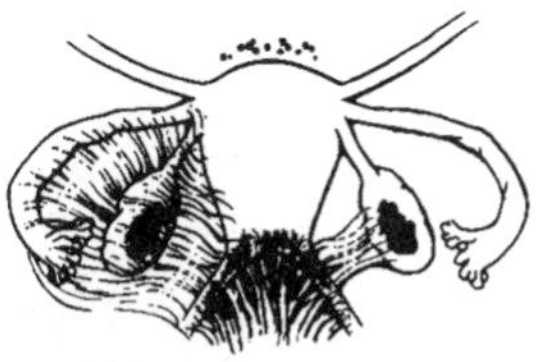

PERITONEUM			
Deep Endo	–	› 3cm	· 6
CULDESAC			
Complete Obliteration			· 40
R. OVARY			
Deep Endo	–	1-3cm	· 16
Dense Adhesions	–	‹ 1/3	· 4
L. TUBE			
Dense Adhesions	–	› 2/3	· 16
L. OVARY			
Deep Endo	–	1-3cm	· 16
Dense Adhesions	–	› 2/3	· 16
	TOTAL POINTS		114

Determination of the stage or degree of endometrial involvement is based on a weighted point system. Distribution of points has been arbitrarily determined and may require further revision or refinement as knowledge of the disease increases.

To ensure complete evaluation, inspection of the pelvis in a clockwise or counterclockwise fashion is encouraged. Number, size and location of endometrial implants, plaques, endometriomas and/or adhesions are noted. For example, five separate 0.5cm superficial implants on the peritoneum (2.5 cm total) would be assigned 2 points. (The surface of the uterus should be considered peritoneum.) The severity of the endometriosis or adhesions should be assigned the highest score only for peritoneum, ovary, tube or culdesac. For example, a 4cm superficial and a 2cm deep implant of the peritoneum should be given a score of 6 (not 8). A 4cm

deep endometrioma of the ovary associated with more than 3cm of superficial disease should be scored 20 (not 24).

In those patients with only one adnexa, points applied to disease of the remaining tube and ovary should be multipled by two. **Points assigned may be circled and totaled. Aggregation of points indicates stage of disease (minimal, mild, moderate, or severe).

The presence of endometriosis of the bowel, urinary tract, fallopian tube, vagina, cervix, skin etc., should be documented under "additional endometriosis." Other pathology such as tubal occlusion, leiomyomata, uterine anomaly, etc., should be documented under "associated pathology." All pathology should be depicted as specifically as possible on the sketch of pelvic organs, and means of observation (laparoscopy or laparotomy) should be noted.

Figure 4.4

Symptoms of Endometriosis

Common Symptoms

- Heavy menstrual periods or other change in menstrual flow
- Severe menstrual cramping
- Painful intercourse
- Infertility

Less Common Symptoms

- Pain in organs outside the pelvic area that worsens during menstruation (e.g., backache, abdominal discomfort, chest pain)
- Constipation; pain and bleeding with bowel movements
- Frequent urinary tract infections; pain and bleeding with urination

---

In the next section, we briefly explore what is known about a new test that may hold a future key to the diagnosis of this disease—a blood test for endometriosis.

Serum Calcium 125

Calcium 125 is an antigen, or protein, that is present in excessive amounts in the blood of 80 percent of women suffering from ovarian cancer. Elevated levels have also been noted in pregnant women and in women with other benign pelvic conditions. Recent work with this chemical marker has focused on its association with endometriosis. Numerous studies now re-

Table 4.1   Classification of Endometriosis

Stage	Points	Findings
I. Mild	1 to 5	Small, scattered, and superficial implants that do not involve the uterus or fallopian tubes; no scar tissue; small, infrequent ovarian implants; no endometriomas
II. Moderate	6 to 15	Multiple, small endometriomas or implants on one or both ovaries; minimal scar tissue formation around the ovaries, fallopian tubes, or other involved sites
III. Severe/	16 to 30	Large tumors of the ovary; extensive scarring with blockage
IV. Extensive	31 to 54	of the fallopian tubes; widespread damage to other pelvic and abdominal structures, including bowel or bladder involvement

veal that the serum obtained from a woman with endometriosis is likely to contain higher levels of Calcium 125 than blood taken from a woman without the condition. More specifically, levels in these women are greatest during menstruation, but don't usually attain the values recorded when ovarian cancer is present. This allows a distinction to be made among cancer, endometriosis, and the absence of any pelvic pathology according to where blood levels fall along a scale.

At present, serum Calcium 125 levels are only in limited use, primarily in diagnosing the recurrence of endometriosis in women who have already had diagnostic laparoscopy and treatment. This is because patients with mild disease have levels very similar to women with no disease. Thus far, abnormal elevations have only been recognized in women with severe disease (Stages III and IV, according to the American Society for Reproductive Medicine classification). However, in the future this ability to differentiate minimal from extensive disease may assist the surgeon in deciding whether surgery is indicated, as well as when a second laparoscopy should be performed to explore a suspected resurgence in disease.

Treatment in the Teen Years

A woman may first experience the pain of endometriosis during adolescence. At this point in her life, dysmenorrhea, more than fertility, is her prime concern. More than likely, she has minimal pathology, and thus minimally invasive therapy may be the extent of any necessary intervention. Still, we must never lose sight of the fact that the seeds of her reproductive future may have already been sown.

In a teenager who has never been sexually active, a clinical diagnosis is often made by performing an abbreviated pelvic exam, palpating the uterosacral ligaments for tenderness and swelling on rectal exam, and performing a diagnostic ultrasound. If signs and symptoms of disease are noted, we must begin management to relieve pain, and more important, to avert any future fertility problems.

Early on, all that may be necessary for pain management are the so-called nonsteroidal anti-inflammatory medications that are both prescription and over-the-counter cousins to aspirin, such as Alleve, Anaprox, Advil, and Motrin. These can reduce the painful effects of prostaglandins to a manageable level, allowing young women with early endometriosis to resume their school life and social activities.

I may also place my young patients on a therapeutic trial of birth control pills. These hormones will effectively prevent spasm, which causes a regression in symptoms. Cycled oral contraceptives really have little beneficial effect on any endometrial implants that may already be present, because as we mentioned before, as long as a woman is bleeding the endometriosis will continue. However, they relieve the dissynergy that exists in susceptible women between the upper and lower portion of their uterus: Normally, when the bottom of the cervix relaxes, the top part contracts. When you have contraction of the lower portion of the cervix, blood may be forced upward into the pelvic structures instead of downward through the vagina. When I place a young woman with severe dysmenorrhea on birth control pills, these agents take over control of the uterus and relieve the spasm via a yet unexplained mechanism. To reiterate, cycled oral contraceptives are not a treatment for endometriosis—they are a treatment for dysmenorrhea borne out of a potential cause of endometriosis and hence may prevent it if Sampson's theory of retrograde menstruation is true.

I try to avoid surgery in adolescents, but if a young woman does not respond to birth control pills, I must resort to laparoscopy to search for the cause of her pain. And if laparoscopy reveals endometriosis, laparoscopic surgery should be performed right then and there.

Treatment in the Reproductive Years— Operative Laparoscopy

Like the other women whose stories we have told in this chapter, Sherry coped with years of agonizing pain from endometriosis. She tells of being rushed by ambulance from her workplace to the hospital one day because the nurse practitioner at the employee health department feared that her appendix had ruptured. In fact, Sherry's excruciating pain was from a large endometrioma located on her right side. She coped as best she could, making do with hormonal treatments and medications because she was unwilling to subject herself to the major surgery she was told would be necessary to eradicate the disease from her body.

All of this changed when she began actively trying to get pregnant. She speaks of that time as being "rescued from an abyss of despair." Sherry decided to see a reproductive specialist who performed operative laparoscopy, excising 90 percent of the endometrial tissue (including a very large ovarian cyst), and repairing one damaged fallopian tube. Now, a year later—pain-free and pregnant with her first child—Sherry says, "I feel like life has started over for me."

Once a woman displaying the symptoms of endometriosis reaches her reproductive years, it is necessary to become more aggressive in the diagnosis and treatment of her disease in order to safeguard her fertility. Specifically, laparoscopy should be performed—both to examine the extent of the disease and to initiate surgical treatment when necessary. The aim of treatment is to contain the spread of endometriosis and to prevent the destruction of the fallopian tubes and ovaries.

The availability of state-of-the-art mechanical tools (such as laparoscopic scissors, graspers, and forceps), laser, and electrosurgery for use in conjunction with laparoscopy may afford the patient an immediate, complete, and low-risk alternative to laparotomy or lengthy courses of drug therapy. Here are some of the advantages operative laparoscopy affords over traditional open abdominal surgery:

- *Same-day surgery, after which recovery time is significantly decreased.* Laparotomy, by comparison, often required a week's stay in the hospital with a three- to six-week recovery time at home. After laparoscopy, women often can return to work in five or six days.
- *Smaller incisions with significantly less bleeding.*
- *Less postoperative pain and infection.*
- *Comparable, possibly even better, results than open abdominal procedures due to better visibility through greater magnification.* Minimally invasive surgery causes less scar tissue, which can be the nidus of a future endometrial implant or a cause of infertility. In addition, the laparoscope offers better visualization of small areas of endometriosis via magnification, thus ensuring a more complete elimination of the disease. It also provides better access to hard-to-reach areas, such as the cul-de-sac (the area between the uterus and the rectum).
- *Less costly.* This is definitely a consideration in today's cost-conscious health care environment.

The Pros and Cons of Using Lasers

Laser laparoscopy has several advantages over traditional surgery: It safely vaporizes and/or excises troublesome implants while cauterizing blood vessels. Less bleeding means better visualization of the operative field, less risk of the need for transfusion, and no need for suturing. As with endometrial ablation, the laser generates heat sufficient to sterilize the wound, cutting down on postoperative infections. But perhaps of most critical importance in endometriosis is that minimal scar tissue is produced during laser procedures. Since adhesions may be the sites of subsequent endometrial implants, such problems are averted in women who have undergone laser surgery. Finally, studies have revealed that laser laparoscopy is highly effective. One such investigation of 158 women noted "Significant relief of dysmenorrhea and dyspareunia as well as enhanced fertility. . . ." In this study, the surgery generally took about an hour and a half, with only four patients requiring hospitalization for observation and none requiring subsequent laparotomy.

Several lasers (including the KTP and nd:YAG types) can be used in the excision and vaporization of endometriosis, but the carbon dioxide (CO_2) laser is the oldest and probably the preferred laser in the excision of endometriosis. This is because its beam may be aimed most precisely over the specific areas to be eliminated and its depth of penetration is minimal. Thus, if endometrial tissue is present on top of a sensitive structure such as the bowel, ureter, or bladder, the CO_2 laser can safely destroy the abnormal tissue without damaging the vital organs underneath. The main problems with the CO_2 laser include that they are expensive, that they are somewhat awkward to manipulate, and that they generate a great deal of smoke, which can interfere with the surgeon's ability to see the operative field clearly. Some physicians who have been well trained in the CO_2 laser continue to use it because it is an excellent tool. I am somewhat leery of the new high-power CO_2 lasers because using them is like speeding in a Ferrari: You have to be very well trained; otherwise you can kill yourself, or worse—hurt the patient.

The newer KTP and YAG lasers have fiberoptic attachments that provide a tangible contact with or a better proximity to the diseased tissue. In addition to their abilities to cut and vaporize, they can also coagulate blood and tissue and thus are more versatile than the CO_2 device. However, because their depth of penetration is greater, the surgeon must take extreme care to avoid damaging underlying pelvic structures.

When I wrote the first edition of this book, the laser seemed to be the best we had to offer women in terms of operative techniques, and lasers are indeed excellent operating tools. But it is to be stressed that the laser is a cutting tool, and it was so popular in the late 1980s because we did not have good tools that mimicked the surgical tools for open abdominal surgery. So we needed a tool with which we could cut, vaporize, cauterize, and coagulate tissue. The CO_2 laser was a perfect source. The problem is that the early lasers were relatively low power, and only recently have we gotten very-high-power lasers that really cut like a knife. Still, the CO_2 laser doesn't cut with the same precision as a knife or even scissors. The KTP, or fiber laser, is more user-friendly for a physician, but it also has a number of drawbacks. The fibers tend to burn up and are expensive to replace. In addition, in cases where the intestines are anchored to the back of the uterus, ovaries, or pelvic side wall, lasers such as the KTP or CO_2 do not offer the flexibility and precision to perform an adequate dissection; thus a sharp pair of scissors and fluid dissection must be used. Lasers have therefore been deemphasized in the last five years, and doctors have begun to treat laparoscopic surgery very much like we treat open abdominal surgery—using scissors and forceps and bipolar coagulators in order to cut and coagulate.

Back to Basics

We have now developed highly sophisticated versions of basic surgical instruments, such as very sharp disposable scissors that do not get dull, better forceps, and graspers, that permit the surgeon to excise endometrial tissue manually. This allows the surgeon to call upon traditional skills and training while keeping costs down. Similarly, special electrical instruments may sometimes be employed to coagulate, cut, vaporize, and/or excise diseased tissue. Electrocautery tools are very powerful and cannot be used to remove endometriosis in very fragile areas of the body.

By now you can see that different devices are appropriate for different types and locations of endometrial tissue. The skilled laparoscopic surgeon will probably use a combination of devices to remove the endometriosis.

Argon Beam Coagulators

Another instrument that I use is the Argon Beam Coagulator, which uses Argon gas to actually blow the blood off pelvic tissues and then shoots a spark out at the tissues to coagulate them. Argon Beam Coagulators are very useful when there are broad areas of endometriosis present in places such as the inside of an ovary. If I find an endometrial cyst inside an ovary, I will first remove the cyst wall and then coagulate the dead tissue, using this instrument because it provides a broad band of coagulation.

AFTER SURGERY, WHAT NEXT?

Unfortunately, neither traditional laparotomy nor modern laser techniques can guarantee a complete and permanent remission for all women. Even though we may infuse a blue dye into the pelvic cavity to try to highlight them, microscopic seedlings or atypical-appearing lesions are sometimes left behind. In my practice, I may institute medical therapy following laparoscopy to prevent the resurgence of any vestigial endometriosis, but it would depend on the degree of the endometriosis and whether the woman desires pregnancy at that time. (In the latter case, medications would be counterproductive.)

Besides oral contraceptives and Danazol, we may now call on an expanded menu of medications that may be rotated to suppress menstruation and ovulation until a woman is ready to become pregnant or until she enters menopause. The following are the major ones used for this purpose.

GnRH Agonists and Antagonists

The use of GnRH agonists in the treatment of endometriosis has been called a "medical oophorectomy" because it effectively shuts down ovarian function and induces a state of pseudomenopause. Many studies now report that women who undergo therapy with these agents experience marked reduction in their implants. Both of these characteristics make GnRH agonists similar to Danazol therapy in some ways. GnRH agonists, however, do not demonstrate the androgenic side effects that 85 percent of women on Danazol complain of—there is no weight gain, acne, deepening of the voice, or hair growth. Perhaps more important, there seem to be no adverse effects on either the liver or on serum cholesterol levels, both of which are known to occur with Danazol.

But the fact that the effects of GnRH agonists are quickly reversible once discontinued is a double-edged sword. On the one hand, ovulation quickly resumes, allowing women to become pregnant almost immediately once their disease has been lessened or eradicated. (Safety in pregnancy is questionable for women while they are on these drugs; therefore, a barrier method of contraception should be used.) It also means that the annoying antiestrogenic side effects, such as hot flashes, decreased libido, and vaginal dryness, are short-lived. On the other hand, this reversibility means that the possibility of an exacerbation of the endometriosis is possible at any time once therapy is discontinued. Long-term therapy with GnRH agonists suppresses estrogen function and thus can cause osteoporosis (see Chapter 9). Because of this, some doctors are experimenting with various protocols of so-called addback therapy.

GnRH antagonists are both similar to and different from GnRH agonists. They are similar in that in the end, their effects on the pituitary are the same. They are different in that agonists potentiate the pituitary's action until it burns out and shuts down estrogen release, whereas antagonists accomplish this directly—immediately affecting gonadotropin release. The main problem with this class of drugs to date has been allergic reactions.

Addback Therapy

With addback or give-back therapy, estrogen and progesterone are given back to women in an attempt to minimize or reverse the adverse effects on bone, the hot flushes, and other antiestrogenic side effects. But no one is quite sure of the proper combinations of drugs needed to prevent adverse effects while still not allowing endometriosis to proliferate. Every woman is different, and for some, even small amounts of estrogen given back might flare up their endometriosis, thus defeating the purpose of the GnRH agonist altogether.

Tamoxifen

Tamoxifen is an antiestrogen medication that may achieve its effect by competing with estrogen for binding sites in target tissues. In limited studies where this drug was administered to women unresponsive to other therapies, tamoxifen showed promise. It seemed to lessen symptoms and shrink implants without causing major side effects. However, some studies have linked tamoxifen to an increased incidence of uterine cancer.

Interestingly, tamoxifen does not always inhibit ovulation and menstruation; thus, pregnancy could occur. Caution: *Do not become pregnant while taking this medication.* Tamoxifen use can cause miscarriages, birth defects, death of the fetus, and vaginal bleeding; it may also cause some of the same problems as DES. Use barrier birth control while taking tamoxifen *and* for two months after you stop taking it.

Megestrol Acetate

Megestrol acetate (Megace) is a powerful progestational drug currently used for the treatment of women with carcinoma of the breast or endometrium. Now it is being introduced as a second-line endometriosis medication, meaning it is prescribed to maintain low estrogen levels and prevent cyclic menstrual bleeding and therefore prevent a recurrence of endometriosis in women under therapy who are not attempting pregnancy. Megace has few side effects except for occasional breakthrough bleeding. It is better tolerated but not as powerful as GnRH in suppressing estrogen.

Gestrinone

Gestrinone (ethylnorgestrienone, R2323) is a steroid that is androgenic, antiprogestogenic, and antiestrogenic. This drug has been used in other parts of the world more commonly than in the United States, and like other medical therapies, it has been somewhat successful in reducing pain and disease, but appears to have no effect on enhancing fertility. In addition, it is not FDA-approved as of this writing.

Synthetic Estrogens and Progesterones

Diethylstilbestrol (DES) is a potent estrogen that gained notoriety a generation ago when a significant increase in the incidence of vaginal cancer was observed in the daughters of women who took this medication during their pregnancies to avert miscarriage. At least two physicians, Drs. Lockhart and Karnaky, writing in the January 1986 issue of the *American Journal of Obstetrics and Gynecology*, have advocated its return from banishment as a treatment for endometriosis, although what its mechanism of action would be is unclear. Presumably, it would compete with the body's natural estrogen for binding sites, as does tamoxifen. According to Lockhart and Karnaky, "Only diethylstilbestrol, properly given, can diagnose the disease without invasion, eradicate endometriotic cells and safely preserve fertility and femininity." This is a controversial area, and the truth of this statement remains to be seen.

Medroxyprogesterone acetate (MPA), otherwise known as Provera or Depo-Provera, is a synthetic progesterone that inhibits the synthesis of gonadotropins. While this medication does reduce signs and symptoms of endometriosis for some women, most physicians believe that more effective medications are now available that cause fewer side effects; however, you will recall that I have had success in some women using this drug in combination with low-dose Danazol.

Both DES and MPA are mentioned here if only to make you aware of their existence, or to clarify information you may have heard about them. They are at this point not the preferred forms of therapy, although they may be used as interim measures.

RU486

RU486 (mifepristone) is best known for its ability to induce miscarriages and is currently under consideration by the FDA for approved use in this country. It is widely used in England, France, and other European countries. RU486 is antiprogestogenic and can interfere with both ovulation and the normal structure of the endometrium. Limited studies and experience with this drug seem to suggest that six-month therapy with it may reduce endometrial pain and implants. If the FDA does follow its advisory panel's recommendation and approve RU486, chances are more data will become available about its effectiveness in endometriosis.

STRATEGIES FOR MANAGING ENDOMETRIOSIS

As I've said before, my management plan for endometriosis depends on the stage of disease that the patient is in as well as her age and plans for childbearing. I prescribe oral contraceptive agents as an initial test for young women with severe dysmenorrhea (painful menstruation). If the oral contraceptive agents work, I will just follow their progress closely. Sometimes I see teenage women with severe dysmenorrhea who may or may not be responsive to birth control pills. If they are responsive, then I will keep them on birth control pills and explain to them and their parents that these pills are beneficial in preventing the full-blown development of endometriosis by relieving spasm. It is very important that these patients be prepared for me to do a rectal examination to check in between the uterosacral ligaments and in the bottom of the cul-de-sac for nodules that are telltale signs of endometriosis. If I find these signs, I then have to proceed to a higher level of treatment. I have to create a state of amenorrhea—the absence of menses. At this time I do a transvaginal ultrasound scan to be sure that there are no endometriomas (collections of endometriosis inside the ovary), because medical therapy will not cure an endometrioma.

The strategy is to make the patient amenorrheic for six months. Initially, I use Depo-Provera and Danazol in combination, and if that doesn't work, I use a GnRH agonist for three months to shut down her cycle and control her pain. (I think it's very important to show women that medicine can control their pain.) Oftentimes after three or four months of amenorrhea and estrogen suppression, I advise therapy with continuous oral contraceptive agents. This will effectively give them back estrogen and help prevent osteoporosis and other problem side effects encountered with several of the endometriosis medications. Most women can continue on non-cycled birth control pills for a year or two to keep their disease under control. Unfortunately, many women choose to stop their medication along the way because they are just tired of taking medication; and then it becomes a constant battle to try to maintain a pain-free and contented patient—sometimes by rotating medications to balance disease progression and medication side effects.

A woman who is more advanced in her disease progression—that is, who is infertile, is very symptomatic, or has big endometriomas—is obviously going to need operative laparoscopy. The goal in operative laparoscopy today is to excise the endometriosis *completely*. A surgeon really must be an expert in operative laparoscopic techniques to try to excise endometriosis. Oftentimes implants lie near vital structures, such as the ureter or the bowel, and sometimes it isn't prudent to excise endometriosis on the bowel. Occasionally, physicians have had to do bowel resections (remove portions of the intestines) where endometriosis has infiltrated—a very difficult situation to deal with.

Oftentimes I will place women with severe disease on a GnRH agonist for a month or two prior to surgery. Although the GnRH agonist sometimes eliminates or shrinks the little seedlings beyond recognition, making them easy to miss, the medical therapy reduces inflammation. Reducing inflammation makes surgery a lot easier, so it's a trade-off. After I perform the laparoscopic repair, I advise these patients to return to GnRH agonist therapy for three months to try to literally dry up the pelvis. Then I will switch them over to either Danazol with Depo-Provera, which will help protect them against osteoporosis, or to continuous oral contraceptive agents. So we have seen that there are a variety of approaches that may be rotated for the treatment of endometriosis.

A common question women ask about these treatments is how long do they have to stay amenorrheic. My answer is that to maximize the potential for childbearing, I prefer to keep them amenorrheic until they are ready to have a child. This duration of therapy ensures that a return of the disease will not mar their fertility. Endometriosis is really an unusual disease, because some people have mild endometriosis that doesn't cause infertility, and there is no evidence that removing endometriosis improves fertility. We do know, however, that if the endometriosis involves and affects the fallopian tubes and the motility of the fertilized egg, the couple is not going to be successful in conceiving a child.

ADENOMYOSIS: ENDOMETRIOSIS TURNED INSIDE OUT?

Margaret is a 52-year-old mother of three who was diagnosed as having multiple fibroid tumors several years ago. She had severe bleeding with her menstrual periods and developed an alarming iron deficiency anemia as a result. In addition, Margaret described the pains she had with her menses as reminiscent of labor contractions. She underwent a myomectomy, and five fibroids were removed from her uterus. Needless to say, Margaret was shocked and dismayed when the surgery failed to have any influence on her pain. It turned out that in addition to the fibroids, Margaret had adenomyosis.

Adenomyosis is also known as internal endometriosis. But this term is only remotely correct in that both endometriosis and adenomyosis are comprised of endometrial glands and stroma present in an abnormal location. The similarities end there. Endometriosis and adenomyosis overlap in only 20 percent of women. Furthermore, adenomyosis more often afflicts middle-aged women (age forty to fifty) who have had several children. In contrast, the most common picture of the endometriosis sufferer is a childless woman in her twenties or thirties.

In adenomyosis, as in endometriosis, the most common symptoms are bleeding and pain. Ectopic endometrium is present, but instead of being located outside the womb, it actually invades the myometrium (muscle layer of the uterus that lies between the outer layer and the endometrium) of the uterus itself. Adenomyosis does not seem to proliferate and bleed cyclically with menstruation as dramatically as does endometriosis. Instead, this aberrant tissue causes a generalized hypertrophy, or enlargement, of the uterine muscle fibers with subsequent overall growth of the uterus. The uterus becomes tender and spongy. Because of this enlargement as well as the pain and occasional abnormal bleeding adenomyosis can cause, it is sometimes mistaken for fibroids.

A definitive diagnosis is difficult to make and is often discovered only after hysterectomy when pathologists examine the uterine tissue that has been removed. Pelvic exam may reveal an enlarged, spongy uterus. Ultrasound and laparoscopy occasionally reveal adenomyosis as well. In addition, MRI is showing promise in detecting adenomyosis as well as in differentiating it from leiomyomas.

In addition to lacking a method of definitive diagnosis for adenomyosis, physicians also lack a definitive form of therapy. For example, adenomyosis has responded poorly to hormonal therapy, perhaps because it seems to be deficient in hormone receptors. Adenomyosis is located in the uterine muscle, making it inaccessible to easy removal. Superficial adenomyosis with abnormal bleeding as its major symptom may occasionally be helped by an endometrial ablation; however, 40 percent of failures of endometrial ablations are due to adenomyosis. Sometimes major collections of adenomyosis in the uterine muscle are identified and removed surgically, either by cutting them out or by performing a technique similar to a myoma coagulation. Treatment is a challenge and is successful in only 60 percent of women who have adenomyosis.

Fortunately, women can have adenomyosis without experiencing symptoms. Unfortunately, for those who suffer its most serious effects, hysterectomy may be their only recourse.

* * *

We have seen that because of the availability of a wide variety of new, less radical treatment options, endometriosis and adenomyosis rarely need to result in hysterectomy. Yet, this does not minimize the detrimental effects endometriosis can impose on women, especially when it strikes during the prime of their careers and reproductive years.

Fortunately, most cases of endometriosis may be successfully managed using a combination of medical and surgical therapies. Women may now undergo one laparoscopic procedure to simultaneously diagnose and treat their disease. Followed up by a combination and/or rotation of analgesics and various suppressive hormonal preparations, their endometriosis may remain in remission for an indefinite period. This permits 90 percent of women to avoid more extensive traditional surgery, including the "routine" initial diagnostic laparoscopy with follow-up laparotomy. The minority of women who do require open abdominal surgery are those whose disease has caused extensive invasion of the bowel. While it is important to note that most times intestinal endometrial scar tissue can be safely separated from the pelvic organs using the laparoscope, most physicians agree that laparoscopic surgery is not feasible if the endometriosis is deeply embedded in the bowel wall.

Although endometriosis continues to present challenges and enigmas, we continue to progress to less invasive and more effective means of helping women to cope with one of the most dreaded "benign" diseases.

Suggestion for Further Reading

The Endometriosis Sourcebook: The Definitive Guide to Current Treatment Options, the Latest Research, Common Myths About the Disease, and Coping Strategies—Both Physical and Emotional, by Mary Lou Ballweg and the Endometriosis Association (Contemporary Books, 1995).

5

HORMONAL IMBALANCE AND DYSFUNCTIONAL UTERINE BLEEDING

In reality, fifteen or twenty days out of twenty-eight (we may say nearly always), woman is not only an invalid, but a wounded one. She ceaselessly suffers from love's eternal wound.
—JULES MICHELET, 1868

In Chapters 3 and 4 we discussed two of the most common organic (structural) conditions that result in hysterectomy—fibroids and endometriosis. However, at some point in their lives, many women experience abnormal uterine bleeding for which no definite pathology can be found, and this can occasionally lead to thoughts of hysterectomy. Copious and erratic vaginal bleeding certainly can be a very frightening symptom and might seem a very logical reason to have an urgent hysterectomy. But as we shall see, this is not necessarily the case. In fact, no surgery of any kind may be needed. Before going any further, it is necessary to understand exactly what is happening when a woman suddenly experiences abnormal uterine bleeding.

A LESSON IN PHYSIOLOGY

Abnormal uterine bleeding is often confused with dysfunctional uterine bleeding. It's important to distinguish between these two conditions. Abnormal uterine bleeding is not a disease; it is a symptom that may signal any one of many different diseases. One well-known text in the field of gynecology, *Jeffcoate's Principles of Gynaecology*, lists over thirty causes of abnormal uterine bleeding, ranging from infections to cancer to heart failure. Thus it is important that your gynecologist considers your entire physiologic makeup and not merely your pelvic organs if you are experiencing unexpected vaginal bleeding. For instance, it may be that your sudden bleeding is a result of a disorder of your hematologic system that interferes with blood clotting, or it may be from a thyroid condition that has altered your metabolism.

Once these disease states have been ruled out, a hormonal imbalance called dysfunctional uterine bleeding is most likely to blame. Dysfunctional uterine bleeding results when there is a disturbance in the normal, cyclical production of hormones by the ovary that may or may not interfere with ovulation. This in turn causes a change in the pattern, duration, or amount of the menstrual flow. It is not a result of another organic cause.

You will recall that every month the brain releases chemical messages signaling the ovary to ready an egg for fertilization. Simultaneously, several follicles housing ova mature, but only one ultimately ruptures; this is called the follicular phase. At the same time, within the uterus, the endometrium is in its proliferative stage, readying itself for implantation should this egg be fertilized. Once the egg is released at ovulation, the ovary enters the luteal phase and the empty follicle becomes a corpus luteum, producing estrogen and progesterone. Within the uterus, the endometrium is now secretory, meaning it is producing nutrients in preparation for sustaining life if pregnancy is inevitable. If no pregnancy occurs, hormone levels decline and the lining breaks down, resulting in menstruation.

The next sections are a bit technical, but please bear with me, because they will explain how and why irregular bleeding comes about.

DYSFUNCTIONAL BLEEDING— THE SHORT MENSTRUAL PERIOD

Sometimes the ovary goes through its normal cycle at an accelerated pace. The follicular phase speeds up for a variety of reasons, as does the proliferation of the endometrium, and menstruation takes place every two to three weeks instead of the usual four to five weeks. This type of dysfunctional uterine bleeding causes more frequent periods without any alteration in the amount of the flow. It may occur after pregnancy while the pituitary is still readjusting, or when any kind of physical or psychological stress influences the nervous system and its subsequent production and release of hormones. This form of dysfunctional uterine bleeding usually resolves on its own in a few months and is no cause for concern.

THE ABNORMAL CORPUS LUTEUM

Another type of dysfunctional uterine bleeding occurs when ovulation takes place normally, but after the release of the egg, the "shell" that remains— the corpus luteum—doesn't function as it should. This condition usually causes heavier, more prolonged periods that come at their normal time. A defect in the corpus luteum in some way causes it to fail to properly produce progesterone, and the endometrium breaks down erratically. While difficult to diagnose, if an endometrial biopsy is performed (to be explained later on), it will reveal an improperly matured uterine lining, a result of inadequate progesterone. More often than not, this is an isolated event. Once the aberrant corpus luteum ceases its activity and the next cycle begins, a woman usually resumes her normal menstrual pattern. Treatment is usually unnecessary unless this tends to happen on a regular basis.

ANOVULATORY BLEEDING

Seventy percent of women with dysfunctional uterine bleeding are at the extremes of their menstrual life (just beginning to menstruate at puberty or just beginning menopause), and 70 percent of women with dysfunctional bleeding are also anovulatory—that is, they do not ovulate. These statistics coincide for good reason, because women most frequently have erratic ovulation either when they are first beginning to menstruate or when they are approaching menopause.

In some forms of anovulatory dysfunctional uterine bleeding, a follicle ripens but no egg is released. Instead, the ovum dies and remains within the follicle, sometimes turning into an ovarian cyst. The ovary produces estrogen, but because there is no ovulation, no progesterone is secreted. This is important because it interferes with the normal functioning of the feedback mechanism that sends signals to the brain to stop estrogen production. Estrogen that is unopposed by progesterone will continue to be manufactured, causing a buildup of the uterine lining that may continue for weeks until the estrogen-producing "granulosa" cells of the ovary literally burn out, like a dying battery. When this finally happens, and when the lining of the uterus has become so thick that the amount of estrogen naturally produced cannot maintain it, the endometrium will begin to break down. A woman who has had no bleeding for perhaps six weeks while estrogen has been building and supporting an unusually heavy lining (called a hyperplastic endometrium) now starts to bleed heavily. This hemorrhaging may continue steadily or erratically for two to eight weeks and can cause serious complications, such as life-threatening anemias.

Interestingly, unlike the severe bleeding that may accompany gynecologic conditions such as ectopic pregnancies or serious infections, dysfunctional uterine bleeding is usually painless, thus providing an important diagnostic clue. Dysfunctional or anovulatory bleeding must be differentiated from more serious conditions such as submucosal fibroids or endometrial cancer. Diagnostic evaluation by hysteroscopy and biopsy is crucial. Dysfunctional uterine bleeding can occur as a result of any disturbance in a woman's physical or emotional state. So delicately in tune are mind and body that menstrual cycles can be altered by physical illness, marital or job-related pressures, alterations in nutritional state resulting in either weight gain or loss, or even "good" stress, such as traveling abroad or moving into a new home. Regardless of the underlying cause, dysfunctional uterine bleeding deserves prompt identification (through the elimination of other pathologic conditions) and intervention to both stop the immediate hemorrhaging and prevent a recurrence.

A DIAGNOSIS OF EXCLUSION

As we've already emphasized, bleeding that appears to be from the uterus may stem from a variety of underlying causes, some of which may not even arise from the genital tract. For example, aside from those disease states elsewhere in the body that may disrupt menstruation, you may perceive that you have vaginal bleeding when the source may be a bladder infection or a hemorrhoid. Because your urethra, vagina, and rectum are in close proximity, it is easy to become confused.

Your doctor should carefully document the source of the bleeding by asking questions about your health history and doing a physical examination, including Pap smear. These are the first steps in establishing the nature of the bleeding. Sometimes, as when the bleeding is a one-time event, careful observation by your doctor may be all that is necessary. If the problem persists, then a physician may order a battery of laboratory tests to check for bleeding disorders, endocrine imbalances, or pregnancy. Transvaginal ultrasound is very effective in assisting doctors in finding the cause of abnormal bleeding because it allows us to examine the ovaries as well as the lining and cavity of the uterus. Ultrasonographic measurements can be taken to determine the thickness of the uterine lining, and this is a vital clue because, for example, if the uterine lining is very thin, cancerous and precancerous conditions of the uterus are less likely. Occasionally, however, hysteroscopy or laparoscopy do need to be undertaken in trying to determine the source of abnormal bleeding. But perhaps the most crucial test in definitively establishing the existence of dysfunctional uterine bleeding is a simple office procedure called an endometrial biopsy.

The Endometrial Biopsy

During an endometrial biopsy, a small plastic cylinder is placed wit
cervix. It contains a device that applies mild suction, allowing a porti
endometrial lining to be withdrawn and sent for laboratory analysis. T
procedure takes only minutes in the doctor's office and causes minima
discomfort.

The cellular structure of the endometrium can tell us a great deal because it normally varies in composition both throughout the menstrual
cycle and when something is awry. (In Chapter 6 we'll discuss the role of
the endometrial biopsy in the diagnosis of cancerous and precancerous
conditions.) If a woman has anovulatory cycles leading to consecutively
missed periods, the endometrium becomes thickly overgrown with tissue—
a condition called endometrial hyperplasia. This is a proliferative endometrium that has not progressed to the secretory phase in many weeks.
The lining has to be rebuilt normally to prevent or stop any abnormal
bleeding and to reestablish a normal menstrual pattern.

THE MEDICAL CURETTAGE

The standard response to dysfunctional uterine bleeding is frequently a
D&C. This effectively removes the endometrium, which may then be
studied for abnormalities. The drawback is that if an underlying hormonal
imbalance exists, this cure is short-lived. It lasts only until the next
anovulatory cycle causes a recurrence of the problem. Unfortunately,
some women have undergone repeated unsuccessful D&Cs, only to wind
up with a hysterectomy when hormonal therapy would probably have
cured their abnormal bleeding without repeated or major surgery!

A medical curettage uses combinations of estrogen and/or progesterone
to shed the uterine lining and allow it to begin anew. It is a simple, safe,
and inexpensive form of therapy that is successful in about 80 percent of
all women. However, it is important to emphasize here that a medical curettage should only be undertaken after endometrial biopsy definitely rules out
any pathology, specifically cancerous or premalignant lesions.

Specific regimens of estrogen and progesterone vary according to the
exact nature of the suspected imbalance and the symptoms you may be experiencing. Your doctor must take care to individualize your plan of care
for your specific condition. For example, if your pituitary gland, ovaries,
uterus, and estrogen levels are all normal but you have missed your
menses, your doctor may suspect that you have failed to produce proges-

ou a course of progesterone to induce your

evere bleeding requires more complex ther-
d ovulation causes nonstop estrogen pro-
a hyperplastic endometrium. Once the ovary
of maintaining the lining with continued estrogen, it
ins, causing profound and unexpected bleeding. Thus it may
necessary to temporarily replace this estrogen and stop the hemor-
rhaging. Afterward, estrogen and progesterone are administered to mimic a normal cycle. Progesterone should convert the proliferative endometrium into a secretory one. Patients need to be carefully monitored over the succeeding months. A repeat endometrial biopsy should be performed to study the appearance of the lining and to ensure that things are indeed back to normal. Once these hormones are withdrawn, a normal menstrual period should ensue.

It's worth mentioning here that other medical therapies have been employed in the treatment of dysfunctional uterine bleeding. They include androgens and androgen derivatives, for example, Danazol, antiprosta-glandins and combination progestins such as Norlutate, and GnRH agonists such as Lupron. All can play a role in arresting or slowing down menstrual bleeding.

In addition, clomiphene citrate, marketed as Clomid, is sometimes used in women with dysfunctional uterine bleeding who desire pregnancy. Clomid induces ovulation and thus reverses anovulatory cycles and the accompanying abnormal bleeding. However, Clomid therapy must be carefully monitored as it can cause some side effects, including the formation of ovarian cysts.

By far, estrogen and progesterone—alone or in combination—remain the most proven remedy for dysfunctional uterine bleeding.

* * *

Dysfunctional uterine bleeding is said to be present when all organic causes of abnormal vaginal bleeding have been eliminated. We now know that it is caused by a problem with the secretion of pituitary and/or ovarian hormones. This sometimes interferes with ovulation and always causes an irregular proliferation and shedding of the lining of the uterus. On occasion, dysfunctional uterine bleeding results in missed periods, but it usually causes excessive bleeding at inappropriate times in the cycle.

In Jeffcoate's most recent edition of his work, *Jeffcoate's Principles of Gynaecology* published in 1987, he advocates hysterectomy as necessary in some cases of dysfunctional uterine bleeding: "In younger women, a radical operation is to be avoided whenever possible but, even in these, there comes a time when hysterectomy with conservation of the ovaries is preferable to incapacity prolonged indefinitely merely for the sake of pre-serving what is likely to be a very unsatisfactory reproductive function." In my view, it is disheartening to see that Jeffcoate has not revised his thinking in over thirty years!

If your doctor suggests a D&C or a hysterectomy, be sure to keep in mind that the many variations of hormonal therapies and the availability of endometrial ablation via either electrocautery or the laser (see Chapter 3) now make D&C outmoded and hysterectomy unnecessary. You should dis-cuss these alternatives with your doctor, and if he or she seems unrecep-tive to these ideas, consider getting a second opinion or changing doctors.

6

THE SPECTER OF CANCER

Hope and patience are two sovereign remedies for all, the surest reposals, the softest cushions to lean on in adversity.
—ROBERT BURTON, 1577–1640

You've watched the scene played on television hundreds of times: The doctor tells the patient, "I'm sorry, Mrs. Jones. You have cancer." The music swells and the drama unfolds; however, we don't imagine that cancer can happen to us. Sadly, cancer strikes in real life thousands of times per year. To be more specific, it was estimated that there were 82,100 cases of pelvic cancer in 1996, resulting in nearly 27,700 deaths (see Table 6.1).

What are your chances of developing a pelvic cancer and what are your chances of surviving it? The figures in Table 6.1 are for the numbers of estimated new cases in the United States for 1996, as well as the survival rates. These numbers are derived from a compilation of data drawn from cancer registries in nine regions across the United States. These numbers have risen dramatically since the 1990 edition of this book, which recorded about 70,100 cases of female reproductive cancer and 23,000 deaths in 1988. One may speculate about the cause of this disturbing rise. Reasons may include the fact that we are an aging population and most cancers occur after age fifty. Other possible explanations may be a corresponding rise in the population and/or better detection methods. Whatever the cause, it behooves us to take a hard look at lifestyle and environmental factors that may afford us the opportunity as individuals and as a society to try to stem this rising tide.

Cancer. Perhaps no other word can so universally conjure up notions of terror. Immediately, we see certain images and have certain questions. Can it be cured? Will I be in pain? Am I going to live? Why me?

As we shall see, not all cancers are created equal. Even within the same organ, cancer can have many faces. This presentation is not meant to be a complete and authoritative discussion of gynecological cancer. Rather, it is designed to introduce you to the wide realm of conditions that are cancerous or can be precancerous. It will leave you with a comprehension of the various treatment options, including hysterectomy.

TABLE 6.1   Cancer Statistics for the United States

Site	New Cases	Survival Rate
Cervix	15,700	68%–88%*
Endometrium	34,000	83%–92%*
Ovary	26,700	44%–76%*
Other and Unspecified Reproductive Cancers	5,700	

*The first (and lower) number indicates the overall five-year survival rate. The second (and higher) figure represents the five-year survival rate when the cancer is detected and treated in its earliest stages.

WHAT IS CANCER?

Cancer is said to occur when the normal replicating mechanism of the cell becomes subverted and abnormal cells grow and develop uncontrollably. Cells, you will recall, are the building blocks of tissue that in turn make up the various organs of the body. Under the direction of genetic material, aging cells are constantly being replaced by fresh, new structures. Although we don't completely understand the entire process, the body normally regulates the extent and timing of these cellular transformations. When there is irregular growth of abnormal cells and these cells physically crowd out the normal tissue and/or alter normal cellular functioning, we begin to notice the manifestations of this process as the signs and symptoms of cancer.

Some cancers grow very rapidly; others are slower. This is generally a reflection of their origin; for example, some tissues of the body have a very slow rate of turnover and cancer cells within that tissue will seem to progress at a slower rate. Because cancer cells lack the inherent protective mechanism of normal cells that tells them when and for how long they should stop reproducing, cancerous cellular growth always overtakes normal cellular growth; for example, even though thyroid tissue and hence thyroid cancer grows very slowly, the cancerous cells quickly crowd out the normal cells. This leads to so much danger and destruction because while cancer cells cannot carry out the life-sustaining functions of healthy tissue, they can and do use up the essential nutrients needed by the remaining normal structures. Sometimes they produce chemicals that disrupt the overall physiology of the body. And while they do die, cancer cells reproduce so quickly that their overall numbers are constantly increasing, never decreasing (unless acted on by outside forces). When cancer cells somehow infiltrate the blood, lymph, or surrounding structures, they quickly extend their path of destruction. This is known as metastasis.

In the following sections, I'll define and describe all the various types of cancer that can afflict a woman as well as those treatments that may allow her to avoid hysterectomy.

CERVICAL CANCER

Cervical cancer is the second most common malignancy of the pelvic organs. One in sixty-three girls born this year will develop it. In most cases, women experience no symptoms, but they may occasionally have some light, irregular vaginal bleeding or a clear, thin discharge. Fortunately, cervical cancer is very slow growing and is 100 percent curable in the earliest stages.

Pap Smears—Who Should Have One
and What Do They Reveal?

A routine test called a Pap smear (see Chapter 2) can usually detect cervical cancer before any significant symptoms appear. Pap tests should begin as soon as a woman becomes sexually active, because, as we shall see, cervical cancer is a sexually transmitted disease. Furthermore, *Paps should continue to be performed throughout a woman's life because, contrary to popular belief, cervical cancer does not cease to be a threat with increasing age or even after a hysterectomy.*

The Pap smear has saved thousands—probably millions—of lives since its development in 1928. Since its introduction into widespread use in 1945, the incidence of deaths from cervical cancer has declined a dramatic 70 percent! However, it is essential to understand that a Pap test is not infallible, but merely a screening test that allows pathologists to examine cells shed from the cervix or uterus. At times, tests will be read as negative because no cancer cells were shed or accumulated on the doctor's spatula when the test was performed. At other times, it may be difficult for a pathologist to pinpoint the exact nature of the problem because the Pap provides only an indirect look at the tissue. Anything identified as a potential concern during the performance of this screening test mandates close and complete follow-up by the gynecologist.

Furthermore, because there might have been some irregularity in the technique of obtaining or reading the slides, many gynecologists (myself included) recommend that women have annual Pap smears. A joint recommendation made in 1988 by the American College of Obstetricians and Gynecologists, The American Cancer Society, and the National Cancer Institute advocates that Pap smears be performed routinely on all women who have become sexually active or those aged eighteen years and up. According to current guidelines of those organizations and institutes, once a woman has had three consecutive negative exams, she may opt to have Paps less frequently depending on her particular risk factors for developing cervical cancer and on other specific circumstances surrounding her individual case. Those organizations believe that *annual* Pap smears may not be necessary or cost effective in every instance because cervical cancer is such a slowly progressive tumor. However, for the reasons I've already indicated, I disagree. I want to emphasize that abstaining from annual Pap smears does not excuse one from a yearly visit to the gynecologist. Annual breast and pelvic exams are crucial to check for other forms of cancer and disease states. It is therefore advisable, in my opinion, to do a Pap test at the same time.

Remember that a Pap smear screens mainly for cervical cancer. Pap tests do not give any reliable information about other forms of cancer, such as that of the uterus or ovary. (Cancer cells from these areas may only rarely reveal themselves on a Pap smear if the disease is fairly extensive and the dead cells have migrated into the cervical canal.)

The cervix is covered with flaky, scaly cells (akin to our skin cells) known as squamous epithelium. Within the os, a different type of epithelial cell is present, known as columnar epithelium. The border where these two types of epithelial cells meet is called the transformation, or transitional, zone. This area is frequently associated with either cancerous or precancerous cells.

Beneath the layer of squamous epithelium are the basal cells—the less mature, rapidly dividing cells that normally should not be present close enough to the surface to be obtained via a Pap smear. Cancerous tissue grows and divides so rapidly that it forces newer or more poorly differentiated cells to within reach of the Pap swab, where they can be detected under the microscope by trained pathologists.

PAP SMEAR CLASSIFICATIONS—WHAT DOES IT MEAN
IF MY PAP SMEAR IS ABNORMAL?

Pap smear classifications today are standardized under the so-called Bethesda System. See the box on page 109.

The Bethesda System describes a number of things about a particular sample. First, it tells whether the sample was adequate. As I mentioned before, sometimes the doctor or nurse practitioner performing the test does not obtain an adequate number of cells, or the patient may have an infection that affects the reading of the slide, etc. The specimen is then placed within a general category of normal or abnormal. Finally, the pathologist

---

Pap Smear Classifications
The Bethesda System: 1991 Revised

The Bethesda System describes the adequacy of the specimen and provides an optional general categorization, such as "within normal limits" or "epithelial cell abnormalities." If the category is not "within normal limits," it will then state "see description" for a more complete explanation of the abnormality. These descriptions, or "descriptive diagnoses," may include such noncancerous cellular changes as a yeast infection or "reactive" changes from a nonspecific inflammation, radiation, or the presence of an IUD. It will then categorize the nature of the precancerous cellular abnormalities, from the least worrisome "atypia" to the most worrisome "severe dysplasias." If the Pap specimen contains noncervical tissue, that tissue is also described; for example, if a vaginal smear is included, the technician or pathologist will note whether the hormonal pattern of the cells is compatible with the patient's age and history (e.g., whether she's postmenopausal or on birth control pills). The following list summarizes the common names or abbreviations given on Pap smear reports under the Bethesda System:

Within normal limits
Benign cellular changes
Infection
Reactive or reparative changes
Epithelial cell abnormalities
Atypical squamous cells of undetermined significance (ASCUS)
Low-grade squamous intraepithelial lesion (SIL)
High-grade squamous intraepithelial lesion (SIL)
Squamous cell carcinoma
Glandular cell abnormalities

---

or technician will describe the cells that are on the slide. For example, the cells on a normal, or negative, Pap test will be described as "squamous metaplasia." Although this might sound ominous, squamous metaplasia indicates completely normal tissue. A slightly abnormal slide may be described as "inflammation."

Perhaps the most confounding classification is "atypical squamous cells of undetermined significance" (ASCUS). This may mean that (as in the case of inflammation) some type of irritant or infection is present that has changed the character of the cells but not in a cancerous fashion. Presumably, the Pap will revert to normal once the cause of the inflammation or infection is discovered and treated. An ASCUS Pap, upon further examination via colposcopy (see page 112)—which should always be done in these cases—sometimes reveals a more significant mild to moderate dysplasia. Certainly, any designations beyond "atypia" or ASCUS are considered to be precancerous or cancerous conditions. Dysplasia or squamous intraepithelial lesion (SIL) are more advanced but still virtually 100 percent curable if caught early.

Cervical Cancer: A Venereal Disease

In the course of researching cervical cancer, some fascinating associations have been revealed. (See the box below.) Demographically, cervical cancer seems to be mostly a disease of the inner city. Although one in sixty-three newborn girls will develop cervical cancer, the risk does not seem to be evenly distributed. Women of lower socioeconomic status are at greatest risk. This is especially true of girls who become sexually active at a young age and who have many partners (especially uncircumcised ones). One theory to account for this is that the transformation, or transitional, zone—an area of the cervix particularly susceptible to cancer—is formed during the teen years. Exposure to many partners during adolescence lends itself to exposure to many infectious agents that may then trigger cancer. How many partners a woman has had and how many partners her boyfriend or husband has had are equally significant. Promiscuous men are more likely to bring home these viruses.

The human papilloma viruses (also known as HPV, condyloma, or venereal warts) have been implicated in precancerous changes of the cervix. HPV may be the most common sexually transmitted disease in the

---

Risk Factors for Cervical or Endometrial Cancer

Endometrial and cervical cancer are the two most common types of malignancies afflicting women, yet the characteristics of the women who develop them are dramatically different. The following list allows you to compare and contrast the risk factors for each, and to examine the steps you can take to lower your risk.

You may be at risk for cervical cancer if you

- Began having intercourse as a teenager.
- Have or had many sexual partners. (*Note:* This also applies if you have been monogamous, but your *partner* has or had multiple sexual contacts.)

- Have contracted certain sexually transmitted diseases, especially genital warts (condyloma acuminata) or HIV.
- Have a partner who has not been circumcised.
- Have a partner who has contracted penile cancer.
- Have been exposed to DES.

You may lower your risk of contracting cervical cancer if you

- Practice "safe sex." In other words, have open and honest discussions with your partner(s) concerning your sexual histories. Get to know the men you are dating, and with whom you are planning intimacy. Use barrier methods of contraception, such as condoms and diaphragms; when used together, these prevent the transmission of venereal diseases.
- Examine yourself (and your partners) for any sores, growths, or discharges in the genital area that may signal a sexually transmitted disease. Seek medical attention promptly if you discover something that concerns you.
- Have annual pelvic exams and Pap tests. Follow your doctor's advice for more frequent exams if you have been exposed to DES or have had an abnormal Pap in the past.
- Practice good hygiene and a healthy lifestyle. For example, women who eat poorly are at a greater risk of developing any kind of cancer.

You may be at risk for developing endometrial cancer if you

- Are overweight.
- Have diabetes or high blood pressure.
- Have had problems with ovulation and dysfunctional uterine bleeding.
- Experienced menopause after the age of fifty.
- Have a family history of endometrial cancer.
- Eat a high-fat, high-cholesterol diet.

You may lower your risk of developing endometrial cancer if you

- Eat sensibly to reduce your weight and dietary intake of fat and cholesterol. Increasing your fiber intake may also be helpful.
- Make good health a priority. See your physician and follow his or her advice to keep blood pressure or diabetes under control.
- Have annual pelvic exams and Pap smears, and report any abnormal vaginal bleeding at once.

United States. Studies reveal that 40 to 70 percent of sexually active women, when tested with special polymerase chain reaction tests available in research facilities, come up positive for HPV infection—oftentimes even when a woman has neither symptoms nor clinical signs of the disease. Men and women may silently pass condyloma between one another, and the end result for some women may be the development of cervical cancer.

Unfortunately, it is not easy to predict whether the mere presence of the virus in a woman's body will be a precursor to cancer. There are over sixty different types of human papilloma viruses—only a few of which seem to have a strong link to cervical cancer. Sometimes the viral infection goes into remission rather than advancing to a precancerous or cancerous state. There might be certain cofactors that make the development of cervical cancer more likely, such as cigarette smoking, stress, the presence of other sexually transmitted diseases, and overall immune status. For example, women who are HIV positive (and thus immunosuppressed) are more likely both to develop a more aggressive case of HPV and to progress to cervical cancer. Cervical cancer in an HIV positive woman is considered to be an AIDS-defining diagnosis. Conversely, it also seems to be true that the presence of HPV in genital tissues compromises them, making them more susceptible to HIV infection.

Other stimuli implicated in cervical cancer include semen and smegma. Among nuns, virgins, and Orthodox Jewish women (whose partners are always circumcised), cervical cancer is almost unheard of. Exposure to DES (diethylstilbestrol) has also been potentially linked to cervical cancer, and more frequent Pap tests are recommended for the women in this category.

The importance of these epidemiologic findings cannot be stressed enough, because they mean that cervical cancer is not only detectable (via Pap smear) and curable, but preventable!

Colposcopy

The next step in the diagnosis of cervical cancer after a suspicious Pap test is a colposcopic examination. This procedure may be envisioned as an extended pelvic exam during which the gynecologist carefully looks at the entire cervix through a microscopelike device. Often, the cervix is bathed with a vinegarlike solution to accentuate the architecture of the cells. Biopsies, or small snips of tissue, are obtained from areas that appear abnormal. In addition, scrapings are obtained from the endocervical canal, the channel within the os that is not visible to an examiner. Experts estimate that colposcopy is 95 percent accurate in detecting cervical abnormalities.

The Cures: Cryosurgery, Laser Surgery, Conization, and LEEP

When cancer cells of the cervix are "preinvasive" (localized), hysterectomy is not necessary. Precancerous changes of the cervix (SIL) may be obliterated by the laser, a loop electroexcision procedure (LEEP), conization, or cryosurgery—all of which are methods of destroying abnormal tissue. Opinions vary as to which method of treatment is preferred for mild dysplasia. In any case, the aim of therapy is to destroy or remove the transformation zone completely. To this end, all four methods offer cure rates of between 90 and 95 percent. Colposcopy and biopsy must precede any type of surgery to confirm the Pap diagnosis, but these procedures are especially crucial prior to cryosurgery and laser surgery because unlike cold knife or LEEP conizations, cryo and laser leave no tissue for postoperative biopsy confirmation. They destroy rather than excise diseased cells.

CRYOSURGERY

An outpatient procedure that does not require anesthesia, cryosurgery involves the application of a cryoprobe, or freezing device, to the cervix to essentially freeze the diseased tissue. Using liquid nitrogen at a temperature of 60 degrees below zero centigrade, the cryoprobe is applied for two three-minute intervals separated by a five-minute thawing-out period. The patient may want to take a mild nonsteroidal anti-inflammatory medication such as Advil prior to the procedure because she may experience menstrual-like cramps. Afterward, she will probably have a watery vaginal discharge for about a month. Other than that, patients experience few side effects or complications. Healing may take up to two months, but there are no scars, no anesthesia risks, no bleeding, and the infection rate is minimal.

I find that the one drawback to cryosurgery is an inability for the surgeon to control the precise width and depth of penetration. The liquid nitrogen used as the freezing material spreads out in all directions and may even bury the transitional zone more deeply, leading to potential problems in following up on any future lesions. In addition, overzealous cryocautery of the cervix can destroy many of the mucus-secreting glands and thereby jeopardize a woman's ability to become pregnant.

Because cryosurgery destroys rather than removes the affected tissue, one would not perform cryo on a suspicious-looking lesion without first waiting for the biopsy report to confirm that the tissue is abnormal. Once cryosurgery is performed, there is no pathology specimen to be sent for postoperative confirmation of the diagnosis; therefore, the doctor must be absolutely certain that he or she is dealing with a suspicious lesion before performing this invasive procedure.

LASER VAPORIZATION

Use of the laser is similar to cryosurgery in that both aim to destroy the transformation zone and both are outpatient, office procedures. However, the laser has the advantage over the cryoprobe in that it can more precisely penetrate and destroy affected tissues. The surgeon has more control over the laser beam, which he or she can direct under colposcopic examination. Laser causes more discomfort than cryosurgery and must be done under local or general anesthesia. Costs are generally higher as well. On a more positive note, healing is cleaner and faster—usually within four weeks.

When more extensive disease is suspected, or when colposcopy fails to confirm the findings of several abnormal Pap tests, it is necessary to progress to a more extensive surgical procedure such as a LEEP or cone biopsy. Both serve the dual role of diagnosing and treating the disease process. Unlike cryo or laser, which destroys the tissue so that postoperative biopsy is impossible because the tissue is unrecognizable, LEEP and conization cut out the tissue, which can then be sent to a lab for analysis.

CONE BIOPSY

During conization, a cone-shaped section of tissue is removed from the center of the cervix. Traditionally done with a scalpel, this procedure is also called a "cold knife" conization. Today, the cold knife is often replaced by a laser or by the LEEP (see below). The cells are then examined to determine how deeply within the epithelial and/or basal layers the abnormalities exist. While diagnostic, the cone biopsy is also therapeutic. In 85 percent of cases, all of the abnormal tissue is removed and the dysplasia (abnormal growth) will not recur. Cold-knife cone biopsy is more invasive than other techniques and cannot be done as an outpatient procedure without general anesthesia. The scalpel can cause bleeding, infection, and permanent damage to the cervix. For example, an overaggressive conization can cause cervical weakness and therefore this procedure carries a risk of miscarriage and infertility. However, cone biopsy is highly effective with a 95 percent cure rate and is still appropriate in certain circumstances.

THE LOOP ELECTROEXCISION PROCEDURE (LEEP)

The newest treatment, the LEEP, is performed by using a fine wire loop that has electrical current passing through it. This current safely removes diseased tissue by cutting and coagulating it. LEEP offers the low cost and simplicity of cryosurgery along with the accuracy, minimal bleeding, and quick cervical healing time associated with laser. In addition, like conization, LEEP removes rather than destroys tissue. Biopsy reports on tissue removed by LEEP occasionally reveal cancerous tissue that would have been missed using cryo or laser surgery. Because of this optimal combination, it is probably the treatment of choice for cervical dysplasia at this time.

Is Hysterectomy Ever Necessary for Cervical Cancer?

Unfortunately, the answer to this question is a resounding YES! The stages of disease categorized as cervical cancer fall along a continuum that we may correspond to the Pap smear classifications already described on page 109. Cellular changes considered to be at high risk of progressing to actual cancer, but which are still precancerous, are the mild and moderate dysplasias grouped under low- and high-grade SIL. These may be treated with laser or cryosurgery with a fair amount of confidence that any further progression to cancer has been arrested.

Squamous cell cancers, sometimes called "carcinoma in situ," may permit conservative treatment with local excision, usually via cone biopsy or LEEP. In this case, carcinoma in situ means that cancerous cells are present but have not penetrated deeply into the layers of the cervix nor invaded surrounding tissues. Naturally, very careful follow-up is necessary for these women to assure that all cancerous cells were excised and have not recurred. Follow-up is also essential to guarantee that the cancerous tissues were genuinely in situ and not invasive.

Truly invasive carcinoma of the cervix must be treated aggressively. "Real" cancer requires "real" treatment—surgery to remove the pelvic organs and nearby lymph nodes to stem the spread of the cancer. Some physicians suggest radiotherapy (destruction of cancerous cells via exposure to strong doses of X rays), but my experience has been that the chance of a successful outcome is greater with surgery. Occasionally, a woman may require radiation therapy prior to surgery in order to shrink extensive tumors so that they are operable. Or she may have radiotherapy after surgery to eradicate residual disease.

While it must be apparent by now that I never resort to hysterectomy when other options are available, with cancer one plays a dangerous game if one tries a "wait-and-see" approach or attempts a partial measure. In the case of a fibroid, for example, it is not life-threatening to attempt to save the uterus via a laser ablation or a myomectomy; if such attempts are unsuccessful, one can always resort to hysterectomy as the ultimate solution. With cancer, there is no such luxury and there may be no turning back. Never hesitate to trade your uterus for your life.

CANCER OF THE UTERUS

Although the uterus is comprised of three distinct layers—the endometrium, the myometrium, and the serosa—the vast majority of uterine cancers grow within the endometrium (the innermost layer). Endometrial cancer is the most common of gynecologic cancers. It will strike one in forty-five newborn girls at some time in their lives, generally when they approach menopause. As with cervical cancer, not all of these forty-five hypothetical newborns have an equal risk (see box on page 110). Unlike cervical cancer, endometrial cancer is demographically linked to the suburbs. In addition, genetic and environmental factors may play a role: This type of cancer tends to develop in certain families, especially among Jewish women and women who eat high-fat, high-cholesterol diets. Associations have also been made between endometrial cancer and obesity, diabetes, and high blood pressure.

But the brightest warning lights flash when a woman suffers from hormonal imbalance of the type discussed in Chapter 5. Abnormal ovulation, prolonged estrogen stimulation, and dysfunctional uterine bleeding are all linked to endometrial cancer. Indeed, they may be precursors in some women.

Hyperplasia

As explained in Chapter 5, a woman may miss several consecutive menstrual periods as a result of hormonal abnormalities that fail to trigger the normal sequence of events leading up to menstruation, including ovulation and surges of estrogen and progesterone. When this happens, the endometrial lining thickens, becoming more and more crowded with glands. This condition is known as hyperplasia. Initially these glands grow in abnormal numbers, but they maintain their normal structure and configuration. Left unchecked, however, these glands possess the ability to grow in abnormal form and progress to cancer.

Any woman with abnormal uterine bleeding, including irregular menses, needs to have an endometrial biopsy. (*Remember*: Pap smears do not screen for endometrial cancer.) Normally, the biopsy will show either a secretory or proliferative lining, depending on the phase of the menstrual cycle. If the endometrium is hyperplastic, treatment must be initiated.

Like cervical cancer, endometrial hyperplasia is a continuum. Cystic and adenomatous hyperplasia are terms for tissue that is still comprised of normal cells but at increasingly high risk of progressing to endometrial cancer. Cystic hyperplasia is rarely of consequence, but 15 to 30 percent of women with adenomatous hyperplasia will develop endometrial cancer in three to five years. With "atypical" adenomatous hyperplasia, there is already some abnormal cell and glandular formation, and cancer is but a step away.

Treatment: Hyperplasia and Beyond

When hormonal imbalance and endometrial abnormalities are detected early enough, they can be reversed rather simply by treatments with potent progesterones. Portions of the lining are initially removed during the endometrial biopsy; then progesterone accomplishes a medical curettage (see Chapter 5) to slough the remaining abnormal tissue. After several cycles of progesterone, the body often resumes its normal functioning and the endometrium reverts to normal.

However, the treatment of adenomatous hyperplasia in this manner must be approached as a calculated risk. Frequent endometrial biopsies are required to assure that there is no recurrence. Abnormal tissue missed on biopsy may mean that the disease may progress to a more serious stage before it is detected and thus require more aggressive therapy than if it were caught earlier. Atypical adenomatous hyperplasia is particularly pernicious. A sixty percent chance exists of developing endometrial cancer. For this reason, oncologists most often recommend hysterectomy for this condition.

As with cervical cancer, cancer of the endometrium requires hysterectomy. The uterus, ovaries, and fallopian tubes should be removed for endometrial cancer. If preoperative tests such as MRI and ultrasound scans reveal an advanced stage, then radical surgery and lymph node dissection with concomitant radiotherapy must be performed. In some centers, radiation therapy in conjunction with surgery is used routinely.

Estrogen and Endometrial Cancer

The earliest forms of birth control pills contained very high doses of estrogen, sometimes without any progesterone present to counteract it. Studies showed that women who took these pills were at increased risk of developing endometrial cancer, and these pills were taken off the market years ago. Some women still have lingering fears about taking hormones, either as oral contraceptives or to reduce the adverse effects of menopause. Recent studies seem to show that hormonal regimens that contain both estrogen and progesterone do not place you at higher risk for uterine cancer and may even lower your risk. (More about this will be discussed in Chapter 9.)

Uterine Sarcomas

Ninety-five to 99 percent of uterine cancers are of the endometrium. However, for completeness' sake, it's necessary to briefly discuss sarcomas: rare malignancies that arise in the muscle or connective tissue of the uterus. (We've already mentioned leiomyosarcomas in Chapter 3.) The prognosis for this type of cancer is guarded at best, and then only if caught in the earliest stages. Treatment options include pelvic surgery with or without radiation and/or chemotherapy.

CANCER OF THE OVARY

When a show business celebrity develops a form of cancer, it is brought to the forefront of public attention through intense media exposure. We may never even have heard of the disease, but suddenly we know its signs and symptoms, its cure rate, and the medical tests we may have been neglecting that may alert us to its presence in our bodies. The death of Gilda Radner, a talented comedienne in her forties, made many women acutely aware of their own risk of ovarian cancer. Fortunately, ovarian cancer is relatively rare, afflicting about one out of every seventy women. A variety of surprising characteristics, from having Type A blood to being resistant to mumps, have been linked to an increased risk of developing ovarian cancer. But a particularly disturbing statistic reveals that women with breast cancer are twice as likely to also develop ovarian cancer and vice versa.

Despite its relative rarity, ovarian cancer is the leading cause of gynecologic cancer–related deaths. Nearly fifteen thousand lives are lost to this dreaded tumor every year. Even more tragic is the fact that the incidence seems to have risen in the past generation, whereas no progress has been made in early detection and cure.

"Silent but Deadly"

Ovarian cancer is called silent because its vague symptoms of abdominal discomfort, bloating, and other mild digestive disturbances might be confused with an entire litany of other medical conditions, from heartburn to gallbladder disease. And it's deadly because the ovary is a very complex organ with a variety of tissue types—all of which have the potential to comprise the "family" of malignancies we know as ovarian cancer. All progress relatively rapidly, and none seem to respond well to the therapies we currently have available. The combination of a cancer that does not generally identify itself until its advanced stages and one that is poorly responsive to treatment adds up to the "silent but deadly" equation.

Yet, no matter how bleak the picture of ovarian cancer seems, it is not a universal death sentence. In my practice I have been very fortunate to have seen very few cases of gynecologic cancers of any type. Francine is one of my few patients with ovarian cancer. She first came to me twenty-two years ago. She is the shining example of never giving up hope despite the odds:

In 1975, when Francine was forty-two years old, she developed pain on her right side that was accompanied by nausea and bloating. She could no longer tolerate the rich foods she had often enjoyed in the past. Her internist initially diagnosed gallbladder disease, but when tests for this condition were negative, Francine was referred to me for further evaluation.

A pelvic exam revealed a suspicious mass on the right side, which was confirmed on X ray. On subsequent surgery, Francine was found to have endometriosis in her right ovary and cancerous tumors in her left ovary. She underwent extensive surgery involving the removal of her uterus, ovaries, fallopian tubes, and portions of her abdominal tissue. This was followed by a two-year course of chemotherapy.

Now, at age sixty-four, Francine is a vibrant and active person. She shows absolutely no signs or symptoms of a recurrence of the ovarian cancer. And while she endured a hellish two years, Francine may now be considered to be cured of her disease.

Diagnosis and Treatment

As mentioned earlier, ovarian cancer is difficult to detect. The symptoms are nebulous and the ovary relatively inaccessible to routine examination. An ovary may have a malignant tumor that is still too small to be evident on pelvic examination. For obvious reasons, Pap smears, biopsies, and so forth are not applicable there as screening tools. Even ultrasound and CAT scans may not be helpful in early diagnosis, although investigation into the use of MRI is progressing. Some blood tests, including ones that monitor liver enzymes, hormone levels, and tumor markers (like serum Calcium 125), offer information regarding the progress of the disease. However, in their present stage of development, these blood tests are not reliable screening tests for the presence of ovarian cancer. Large-scale investigations using serum Calcium 125 and/or vaginal ultrasound failed to detect ovarian cancer in its early and thus more treatable stages. Therefore, such screening methods are controversial, and some doctors believe that they are really of value only to women who are at high risk, such as those with relatives who have had ovarian cancer. Some doctors now recommend screening vaginal ultrasound examinations for women in their late reproductive and menopausal years. Women who appear to have significant ovarian cysts on sonogram and women who have any cancer symptoms, such as they are, should have frequent ultrasound examinations. Although imperfect, at least this technique offers some chance at early detection. And any woman over forty with an ovarian cyst that does not resolve in a few menstrual cycles must have an exploratory laparoscopy or laparotomy. The extent of the surgery depends on the size, the nature, and the degree of suspicion a particular ovarian tumor possesses.

As one might imagine, the treatment of ovarian cancer should be as aggressive as the disease. It frequently involves removal of the pelvic organs along with the appendix and portions of the intestinal covering known as the omentum. In addition, radiation and chemotherapy are often employed as adjuncts to surgery.

CANCER OF THE FALLOPIAN TUBES

Cancer of the fallopian tubes is one of the rarest of all cancers. In fact, most gynecologists will never see a case during their entire careers. It afflicts one of every thousand women, but because of its rarity, no epidemiologic statistics exist to identify women who may be at higher risk for developing it. While it has been suggested that chronic inflammation of the fallopian tubes may be a precursor, this is difficult to pin down, since there are so many cases of salpingitis (inflammation of the oviducts) as compared to so few cases of cancer.

Although a myriad of symptoms may be associated with this type of malignancy, none is characteristic or dramatic enough to raise the red flag. For example, a woman might have vaginal bleeding, pain, or discharge. She may feel a sense of pressure or bloating in her abdomen. A mass may be felt during a pelvic examination. All of these may be symptoms of other, more common forms of cancer or other noncancerous conditions, such as pelvic inflammatory disease or ectopic pregnancy (a pregnancy that develops in the fallopian tube rather than the uterus).

The treatment and prognosis of fallopian tube cancer unfortunately follow along the same lines as ovarian cancer. Difficult to detect in its earliest stages, this cancer is rapidly progressive and destructive. Surgery and radiation are utilized to attempt to eradicate the malignant tissue.

CANCER OF THE VULVA AND VAGINA

We began this chapter with a cancer that is frequently preventable and curable and we can end with one as well. Cancers of the vulva, like cervical cancers, seem to have links to human papilloma viruses. Poor hygiene practices may allow these infectious, potentially precancerous irritants to remain on the surface of these structures, thus opening the door to cancer. However, unlike cervical cancer, these malignancies are very rare (only slightly more common than fallopian tube cancer) and almost always strike women in their late sixties and early seventies.

Finally, we have vaginal cancer. Only five women in one million develop vaginal carcinoma, and as with vulvar cancer, these women are well past menopause. The significant exception to this rule are the daughters of women who took DES (diethylstilbestrol) during their pregnancies to avert miscarriages. These DES daughters develop vaginal cancers early in life. (The peak incidence seems to be at about age nineteen, with about one out of every thousand women affected.)

Although cancers of the vulva and vagina are rare, easily detectable, and highly curable in the earliest stages, a criminal number of women die from them every year. This can be attributed only to ignorance and negligence. Older women and their doctors may omit Pap smears and pelvic exams, believing them to be unnecessary, uncomfortable, and embarrassing when a woman is "so old," is no longer sexually active, or may even have had a hysterectomy. They forget that these women are in the highest risk group.

Both vulvar and vaginal cancers are susceptible to a variety of treatment options falling short of hysterectomy, including laser surgery, cryosurgery, and treatment with radiation or topical chemotherapeutic agents.

* * *

Thousands of hysterectomies are performed in the United States every year for gynecologic cancer. Most are justified. Once a flagrant malignancy has developed, nothing short of its total obliteration may be attempted at the risk of a woman's life. However, I'd like the emphasis here to be on the positive—the potential for prevention and minimizing one's risk of developing a cancer in the first place.

We've seen that certain cancers, such as those of the cervix, vulva, and vagina, are linked to certain diseases and irritants. Women can avoid these by taking commonsense precautions, including practicing good hygiene, using condoms, and having regular Pap smears. Other cancers seem to be more common among women who are obese, because fat stores estrogen. So-called estrogen-dependent cancers include cancers of the breast, ovary, and endometrium. It is therefore no surprise that eating a diet low in fat and cholesterol as well as high in fiber will decrease the risk of developing ovarian and endometrial carcinomas.

But even after decades of research, so much about cancer—its causes and cures—remains a mystery. Sadly, as we continue to pollute our environment and expose ourselves to so many potential carcinogens in air, water, food, homes, and workplaces, cancer rates mount. It is difficult to say what is ultimately responsible for these frightening statistics. Perhaps it is environmental factors or the mere fact that a century ago women died of infectious diseases or childbirth long before their cells aged enough to mutate into cancer. Most likely, it is a combination of many factors, including genetic makeup as well as exposure to toxins.

While we each may have some risk factors that we cannot change, we can all make an impact on many other risks. Women currently have the edge over men when it comes to cancer deaths—perhaps because women smoke less (although this is changing), drink less, seek medical care on a more regular basis, and have less occupational exposure. Let's hope that women do not fall behind in the battle against cancer. A healthy lifestyle that includes a nutritious diet, a minimum of stress, sound medical care, and a safe environment will keep women's immune systems in top fighting shape to do battle against the cancer foe . . . and to win.

Major Signs and Symptoms of Pelvic Cancer
See your doctor if you notice any of the following:

- Any unusual growths or sores on or near your vulva. The genital warts (condyloma, HPV) that seem to be linked to cervical cancer look like flesh-tone cauliflowerlike pimples; they may appear singly or in clusters and are painless. Vulvar cancers appear as raised sores or ulcers that are painful, may ooze or bleed, and don't heal.
- Vaginal discharge.
- Abnormal uterine bleeding. Any change in the normal flow; that is, a change in the amount, duration, consistency, or timing of vaginal bleeding.
- Spotting after intercourse.
- Palpable lumps in your abdomen, noticeable bloating, or increase in abdominal girth.
- Abdominal pain, nausea, vomiting, gas, constipation, weight loss, or loss of appetite.
- Swollen glands in the groin area.
- Painful, frequent, or difficult urination.

7

UTERINE PROLAPSE
AND URINARY
INCONTINENCE

To cure sometimes, to relieve often, to comfort always.
—ANONYMOUS

Up to 1990, the most recent year for which nationwide hysterectomy statistics are available, prolapse of the uterus accounted for 16 percent of all hysterectomies performed. Today, it is often unnecessary to go to the extreme of performing a hysterectomy when other techniques—both surgical and nonsurgical—can provide a solution to this common condition.

PROLAPSE—HERNIAS
OF THE PELVIC FLOOR

The uterus, vagina, bladder, and rectum are all attached to the pelvic walls by a network of muscles, nerves, and blood vessels called the pelvic diaphragm. Prolapse is the term used to describe what happens when weakened support structures (connective tissue) allow the uterus to descend from the pelvic cavity into the vagina or the vagina itself to turn inside out and drop toward the vulva. This weakness actually represents a hernia formation. Weakness in the supporting tissues, either from childbearing or tearing of tissues due to stress (as, for example, from ballet dancing or aerobic exercise), allows descent of the uterus into and out of the vagina. When the uterus prolapses, it drags with it the upper portions of the vagina, and in rare, severe cases, the entire cervix and uterus protrude entirely outside the body.

Prolapse has been recognized from earliest times, and it's interesting and amusing to read how my physician predecessors accounted for this condition. For example, both the ancient Egyptians and the ancient Greeks believed that the uterus had a personality all its own, and therefore could move about independently and at will. Thus if it were attracted to something outside of the body, the uterus might migrate toward it.

Centuries later, the Victorian Age brought yet another "explanation." Prolapse, it was believed, came about when a woman engaged in activities she really wasn't designed for, such as singing, dancing, horseback riding, skating, wearing dresses with tight lacings, and worst of all—masturbation! Truthfully, Aretaeus, a Greek physician who lived during the second century A.D., was probably more on target when he blamed strenuous labor as a cause of prolapse. Victorian women were certainly more at risk of developing a prolapsed uterus from the obstetrical practices of the time as well as from their physical labors than from singing or skating.

Still, uterine prolapse through the ages has been a common affliction, especially for older women. Although prolapse accounts for 16 percent of hysterectomies overall, this figure becomes almost 40 percent in women over age sixty-five. In other words, four out of every ten women undergoing hysterectomy after age sixty-five do so for uterine prolapse. But is hysterectomy always necessary?

Thirty years ago, we often used mild prolapse of the uterus to justify a hysterectomy to a hospital committee that would otherwise have required a woman to have as many as six children before she could be sterilized. We'd place an instrument on her cervix, and attempt to pull it down into the vagina so as to be able to say that she had a so-called uterine prolapse with traction. Fortunately, these tactics are considered to be unnecessary and unethical today, when no woman should have a hysterectomy suggested to her solely for sterilization purposes. Very few women—even those who do have legitimate prolapse—require hysterectomy today.

What Happens

Think of a prolapse as a hernia or bulging of tissue that occurs within the vagina. The uterus, vagina, bladder, and rectum are all held in place by a unified system of supporting ligaments, muscles, and other tissues that resemble a sling. When a weakness develops in these structures, there will be a sagging of this sling that in turn causes a protrusion into the usually taut vaginal wall.

Normally, only a small portion of the neck of the uterus (the cervix) is present at the very top of the vagina. As already mentioned, if its support structures loosen, the uterus will then drop down further into the vagina by virtue of its weight and the pull of gravity (see Figure 7.1). The uterus cannot prolapse without carrying portions of the vagina along with it and thus causing a "vaginal prolapse." (When the uterus falls, it literally turns the vaginal wall inside out.) But the vagina can prolapse independent

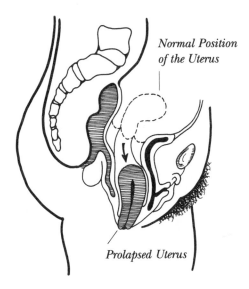

Normal Position of the Uterus

Prolapsed Uterus

Figure 7.1 *Uterine prolapse*—The uterus drops down into the vagina due to weakening of its support structure.

of the uterus and, in doing so, can affect bladder or bowel functions. Fortunately, vaginal vault prolapse is rare, affecting no more than twelve hundred women in the United States annually.

When a weakness in the vagina occurs in its upper portion, the bladder (which lies directly above the vagina) may lose its "footing" and drop down so that it is bulging into the vagina. This condition is called a cystocele. (If only the urethra, or tube through which the urine actually exits the body, is involved, this is known as a urethrocele.) If, however, the weakness develops in the lower wall of the vagina, loops of intestines (an enterocele) or the rectum itself (a rectocele) may protrude into the vaginal walls.

Why It Happens

The direct cause of these conditions is not entirely clear, although certain factors are known to increase the likelihood of developing a prolapse. Pregnancy and childbirth are most frequently implicated. But let's look more closely at these so-called predisposing factors.

Interestingly, when women with known uterine prolapse become pregnant, it is usually only in the earliest stages of pregnancy that their condition is aggravated. Once the womb enlarges, it rests on the pelvic brim and is kept from descending further into the vagina. Therefore, contrary to popular belief, pregnancy probably does not cause or exacerbate a uterine prolapse.

Labor is another situation entirely. A prolapsed uterus is rarely seen in women who have delivered only via cesarean section. But what is puzzling is the observation that some women can endure multiple or extremely traumatic births without ever developing a prolapse, whereas other women need never have had a child to develop prolapse. Clearly, other factors are involved.

A strong family history seems to be associated with this condition. Some women are genetically prone to develop a prolapse due to an inherent weakness of the muscles and tissues that support the uterus and vagina. It is particularly important for susceptible women to have expert obstetrical care to avoid events that might trigger a prolapse. For example, while women these days are anxious to avoid episiotomies (a small surgical incision made in the perineum to enlarge the vaginal opening to accommodate the baby's head), they may be inviting prolapse at a later date by sustaining unseen muscular tears and other injuries from excessive and prolonged efforts at delivery. Thus the desire to avoid an episiotomy must be balanced by the desire to avoid future prolapse. Furthermore, you can help to minimize the risk of childbirth-related prolapse by doing Kegel exercises (see page 132) and avoiding constipation during and after your pregnancy.

It's important to realize that women can, but usually do not, develop prolapse immediately after giving birth. It is perhaps during that period of time when the weakness first develops; however, it is generally years later, as menopause approaches and estrogen levels decline, that the actual prolapse occurs. It is believed that estrogen helps to maintain the muscle tone and blood supply to the pelvic structures and thus prolapse and/or urinary incontinence, a common symptom of prolapse, will occur once estrogen levels decline.

Ironically, hysterectomy may be both the cause and the cure of a vaginal prolapse! In some cases, the surgical removal of the uterus, especially when it is performed via the vaginal route (see Chapter 8), can cause a weakness in the vagina resulting in subsequent vaginal vault prolapse. If the surgeon is not careful in his or her technique, a woman may need another operation to repair and strengthen the vagina posthysterectomy. As many as 40 percent of women having hysterectomy subsequently experience some degree of vault prolapse.

WHEN DO YOU NEED HYSTERECTOMY?

Hysterectomy can be avoided in many cases of uterine, vaginal, bladder, and rectal prolapse. Young women who develop a prolapse can have the supporting structures repaired. It has been traditionally said that if the

---

Symptoms of Uterine Prolapse

- A fleshy protrusion that is palpable inside the vagina or visible outside the vagina, especially when you strain, cough, or laugh.
- A sensation of fullness, heaviness, or pressure within the vagina or in the lower abdomen.
- Frequent bladder infections, with associated burning pain, urge to urinate, more frequent urination, urinary retention, and/or blood-tinged urine.
- Leakage of urine or feces with sneezing, coughing, laughing, or straining (stress incontinence).
- Bowel movement disturbances, such as difficulty in moving your bowels or completely emptying your rectum.
- Lower back pain.

---

uterus is left intact, it acts as a piston that will cause the prolapse to recur, but I don't believe that's necessarily true. In the majority of cases, whether you need a hysterectomy or even a prolapse repair really depends on the severity of the prolapse and how uncomfortable you become as a result. In other words, because a prolapse is never a life-threatening condition and very rarely causes even a serious problem, the best advice is, Don't bother it if it doesn't bother you. The next question is, how might it bother you? (See box above.)

Naturally, the symptoms depend on the structures involved. Slight uterine prolapse is rarely noticeable. As the uterus protrudes further, you might feel a sensation of heaviness, dragging or fullness in your vagina or lower abdomen. Medical intervention (but not hysterectomy) is necessary only when the cervix and/or uterus actually protrude from the vulva, because they may develop infected sores from the irritation of being exposed to the outside.

TAKING CARE OF PROLAPSE

Remember that a cystocele is a condition in which the bladder drops down and bulges into the vagina. But before we discuss the problems and solutions that encompass cystoceles, it is necessary to explain how the bladder normally works.

The urinary tract consists of two kidneys, which filter out waste products from the bloodstream as it circulates through them and manufactures urine; two ureters, which are pathways that connect and transport urine to the bladder; the bladder, which stores urine before it is eliminated from the body; and the urethra, the spout through which the urine is expelled. In order for urination to occur, the neck, or sphincter, that lies at the bottom of the bladder must relax while the bladder itself contracts. A unique muscular sling called the posterior urethrovesical angle lies beneath the urethra at the junction of the bladder and the urethra. This sling of tissue can actually be traced all the way up to the back of the pubic bone. During periods of stress the sling normally tightens, and in order to urinate, you must consciously relax the sling. The bladder is then compressed and expresses the urine past this sling of tissue. Weakening of this sling results in an increased ability of the bladder to move up and down and side to side. The sling loses its ability to pull up on the urethra (the spout), and in periods of stress, such as coughing, laughing, and sneezing, or during participation in certain types of athletics, some urine will leak. This condition is called stress incontinence.

Researchers find stress incontinence to be as common in women without prolapse as in women with prolapse. Furthermore, the surgery involved in correcting uterine prolapse may actually contribute to stress incontinence and, at best, may not correct it. More specifically, a uterine prolapse or a cystocele doesn't automatically result in losing control of bladder function. A cystocele is purely an anatomical defect and is sometimes completely symptom-free. You do not need and should not have surgery to correct a symptom-free cystocele unless you're looking for trouble. Attempts to suspend the bladder oftentimes reduce the posterior urethrovesical angle (the connection between the bladder and the urethra)—the angle that allows the neck of the bladder to contract. This alteration in anatomy can contribute to recurrent stress incontinence after prolapse surgery. Therefore, it is important that the surgeon always leaves a little bit of a cystocele in order to prevent the straightening of this angle.

Today, most of the surgery for stress incontinence involves not only pushing up the bladder or making a stronger cuff to support the bladder (in what is called the Kelly plication technique), but also a Burch procedure, in which the tissues alongside the connection to the bladder and the urethra (the posterior urethrovesical angle) are suspended and hitched to the back of the pubis or to the thick fibrous tissue (Cooper's ligament) that lies in the back of the pubic bone. (See Traditional Surgeries—Vaginal Repairs for more details.) This procedure is quite successful and can be done either by open abdominal surgery or by laparoscopic techniques.

If you have a prolapse that seems to be causing stress incontinence, you need to have a series of tests called cystometric studies (bladder muscle tone studies) to ensure that the incontinence is not from a neurological problem or other physiologic cause requiring medical, not surgical, intervention. These tests measure the bladder capacity and the competency of the nervous system that allows the sling to constrict or relax. Urologists can also measure the ability of the bladder to contract its upper portion and to relax the sphincter and allow urination to proceed in a normal matter. If this test is not done, you run the risk of having major surgery to correct a problem that is not surgically correctable.

You should be very skeptical of surgery meant to reverse stress incontinence, and you certainly need to undergo thorough testing for other underlying urinary conditions before consenting to surgery—lest you be bitterly disappointed with the results.

Besides stress incontinence, cystocele may rarely cause other conditions that necessitate surgical repair (but not necessarily hysterectomy). The bladder is shaped somewhat like a horizontal balloon with a "neck" at its base ending in the urethra. Sometimes with a cystocele, the balloon portion of the bladder drops down lower than its neck, thus impeding the flow of urine. In such cases, you may have difficulty emptying your bladder. As a result, you may constantly feel the urge to urinate, but may be able to eliminate only small amounts. Eventually, as urine accumulates in the bladder, you may develop frequent infections causing painful urination.

Various approaches are used to repair a cystocele, including lifting the bladder from above through an incision in the abdomen, or opening the vaginal wall and pushing up the bladder from below. Unfortunately, even under the best circumstances, cystocele repairs are not a guaranteed cure, since the weakness of the tissues can return. Thus, before considering surgery for a cystocele causing stress incontinence, you should try to alleviate your symptoms by strengthening your tissues with exercises and/or estrogen replacement therapy.

Hysterectomy need accompany cystocele repair only when the uterus itself is also significantly prolapsed. If this is not the case, adding hysterectomy to cystocele repair only makes the surgery and its aftermath more complicated. Unfortunately, in many cases the supporting tissues that have weakened to allow bulging of the bladder into the vagina have also caused the uterus to drop down. Repairing a very severe prolapse may require removal of the uterus. This is because in these cases the uterus acts like a piston that pushes down in response to abdominal pressure. The uterus has the potential to prolapse again, necessitating repeated surgery.

A rectocele—a condition in which the rectum protrudes into the weakened vaginal wall—is usually asymptomatic and little cause for concern. Women with rectoceles may complain of backaches, but there is usually an underlying cause of the back pain that is unrelated to the rectocele. The main problem with a rectocele may be difficulty in defecating and completely emptying the rectum. Interestingly, a previously "silent" rectocele may suddenly become troublesome once the uterus is removed, so hysterectomy should never be suggested for this reason. If hysterectomy is necessary for another cause, it's important that any large rectoceles also be eliminated at the same time.

TRADITIONAL SURGICAL INTERVENTIONS—VAGINAL REPAIRS

A vaginal repair is done to correct a cystocele, rectocele, and vaginal prolapse. During a vaginal repair, the surgeon dissects the vaginal tissue, exposes the bladder and urethra, and then folds over the tissue to create new support for the posterior urethrovesical angle. Vaginal repairs may cause more problems than they cure. They may lead to sexual difficulties (such as painful intercourse), particularly if the vagina has been surgically narrowed or shortened. As mentioned earlier, they may also cause or worsen stress incontinence. It is most important to determine the true cause of urinary leakage.

True stress incontinence stems from a hypermobility of the urethra, and can be demonstrated on ultrasound examination. Surgery is then employed to anchor the angle between the urethra and bladder and prevent the involuntary leakage of urine. If the bladder is prolapsed but the urethra is fixed, you won't have any incontinence. If there is a hypermobility of the bladder and urethra, it is necessary to put sutures alongside the angle between the bladder and the urethra and then attach it to Cooper's ligament, which is a very strong fiber and would solidly hold all the structures in place and prevent any stress incontinence. This is called a Burch operation.

This surgery was traditionally performed via an abdominal approach. In other words, we had to make an incision and dissect, tunnel down under direct vision into this area alongside the bladder, elevate the bladder, and do the suturing I described in an operation called a Marshall-Marchetti procedure. This operation and the Burch procedure can now be performed laparoscopically. Laparoscopic surgery affords all the advantages we have previously talked about in this book, but it is imperative that anyone desiring a laparoscopic correction of prolapsed tissues seek an expert in these techniques, because placing these sutures via the laparoscope is very difficult to accomplish.

MODERN SURGICAL TECHNIQUES— SACROSPINOUS FIXATION

Sometime in the last ten years, doctors began putting stay sutures (permanent sutures) into the vaginal vault tissues after hysterectomy to prevent prolapse from occurring postoperatively. This is an old operation, but new techniques have repopularized the procedure. They also began placing these special sutures in the vaginas of women who already had some prolapse and wanted to avoid hysterectomy. Because these stay sutures are fixed to the sacrospinous ligament, this operation is called a sacrospinous fixation. Here's the clearest analogy I can draw for you to help you picture this procedure: Imagine putting in stakes with attached ropes at three or four points on a lawn, then attaching the ropes to a tree for the purpose of holding up that tree. The sacrospinous ligament is a very strong ligament that may be used to anchor the pelvic structures and prevent prolapse in much the same manner as stakes can anchor a tree.

Twenty years ago, urinary incontinence was treated by repairing a cystocele vaginally. In contrast, today we do a lot of procedures that pull up the bladder and actually fix it to Cooper's ligament, which lies right behind the pubic bone. As a result of these modern techniques, we have a far better success rate now than we did in the past. So today when a woman is suffering from urinary symptoms and prolapse, we try to plan our surgical procedure to usually include a posterior urethral suspension. We know that the first repair is always the best repair, and if the surgeon does a poor vaginal-type repair, there is almost a 50 percent chance that in five years it will break down.

TREATING URINARY INCONTINENCE WITHOUT HYSTERECTOMY

As mentioned briefly before, the most common symptom of prolapse of the bladder, uterus, or vagina is the involuntary loss of urine, known medically as urinary incontinence. As many as a quarter of all women under age sixty, and up to 30 percent over age sixty, suffer from this symptom, but less than half seek medical help for their problem, probably due to embarrassment. This is tragic because urinary incontinence can cause many complications, including social isolation, loss of sexual desire and decreased sexual performance, hygiene problems leading to urinary tract infections and skin irritations, and depression. Yet its cause—a medication side effect or a urinary tract infection—may be easily reversible. A woman going to her doctor for urinary incontinence should *never* be told she needs a hysterectomy until all nonprolapse-related causes have been ruled out and other less invasive treatments have failed. A neurologic (nervous system) or endocrine (hormone-related) cause may be found, in which the answer is bladder training or medication—not surgery.

Self-Help

We already know the multitude of problems that hysterectomy can cause. Most are not worth risking for the relatively simple and benign condition of a prolapsed uterus, unless it is truly hindering the quality of your life, and even then laparoscopic procedures can repair pelvic tissues without removing them. In addition, you should try various nonsurgical approaches before resorting to surgical intervention.

KEEPING TRACK OF INTAKE AND OUTPUT

All incontinent women should limit the amount of fluids that they drink—especially caffeine and especially at night. As a general guide, I recommend not exceeding the equivalent of a two-liter beverage bottle per day or more than eight ounces of coffee, tea, or soft drink per day. If you are incontinent, you should also try to empty your bladder frequently.

Keep a diary of your bathroom habits for a day or two. This information can be reviewed by a doctor or nurse with the goal of helping to establish a diagnosis, and if appropriate, a program of bladder training can be designed to assist you in returning to a more normal pattern. The diary should include:

- When and how often you urinate
- How much urine you are producing
- Whether you have been incontinent (including any bedwetting) and when
- Whether you get up at night to urinate
- How much fluid you have had
- Whether you have had any unusual symptoms, such as burning with urination, feeling the urge but being unable to urinate, etc.
- Whether you are on any medications, because some will increase urine production and/or affect bladder control

KEGEL EXERCISES

A California physician named Dr. Arnold Kegel developed these exercises to help women to strengthen the muscles of their pelvic floor. While they are fairly simple to learn and can be performed virtually anywhere, like any exercise, they require persistence and perseverance to obtain successful results. A stronger pelvic floor not only might improve the symptoms of prolapse and stress incontinence, but also frequently enhances sexual pleasure and helps younger women to prepare for childbirth. Here's how they are done.

You must first locate the exact muscle group you need to work on. To do so, try to stop and start your stream of urine, or alternatively, attempt to squeeze your partner's penis during intercourse. The muscles you use in these attempts are the ones you need to strengthen.

Contract, or tighten, these muscles for two or three seconds, and then relax them in an alternating pattern of contraction and release for a cycle of ten repetitions. Gradually increase the number of cycles you perform each day until you are doing twenty groups of ten Kegel exercises. This may take a month or two to work up to. Remember that you can do these exercises while you are otherwise engaged, whether you are standing on line in the bank or sitting at your desk in the office.

Biofeedback can be used in conjunction with bladder training and Kegel exercises to improve the outcome. For example, a woman who has difficulty pinpointing the correct muscle groups can get a visual or auditory signal to tell her when she's performing the exercises correctly and to reinforce her attempts.

Nonsurgical Treatments

A variety of vaginal devices or medications are available to treat urinary incontinence. Here are some of the most common ones.

PESSARIES

If you are unwilling or unable to undergo surgical repair of a uterine prolapse, a pessary may be the answer. This is a device made of plastic or rubber that fits firmly in the vagina and physically supports the uterus. Pessaries come in a variety of models, including ones that are inserted into the vagina and then inflated with a small air pump as well as ones that are of a fixed size and shape. A pessary does not cure prolapse; it merely holds up the tissues. It may be inconvenient for you if you are active or frequently engage in intercourse. Likewise, if you are in poor health, you may find a pessary cumbersome to insert or uncomfortable to wear. However, it is certainly a simple solution, free of the complications of surgery. For Millie, it was the answer to her prayers.

Millie is a vegetable farmer who is on her feet many hours of the day. At age 62, she leads an active life, which includes not only physical labor, but attending to her husband and six grandchildren. She does not desire surgery for her uterine prolapse, but instead uses her pessary as needed to avert discomfort. She inserts it and removes it at her convenience.

Pessaries may also be ideal for you if you experience stress incontinence only with vigorous exercise. Insert the pessary (or a diaphragm or tampon) just prior to your workout and remove it afterward.

Not every woman will elect to use a pessary. If you have significant symptoms from vaginal or uterine prolapse, and you prefer the surgical solution over exercising or dealing with a pessary, that is perfectly acceptable. The key here is that the choice is yours and not your physician's.

VAGINAL CONES

The vaginal cone is a tamponlike device that comes in a variety of weights. The aim of therapy is to train the muscles to retain the greatest amount of weight possible within the vagina for fifteen minutes twice daily. Like Kegel exercises, the pelvic floor muscles will become progressively stronger with increasing weight, thus allowing you to retain urine more effectively.

ELECTRICAL STIMULATION

Functional electrical stimulation devices trigger mild nerve stimulation to cause contractions of the pelvic floor muscles, toning them and again decreasing incontinence. The electrical impulses are conveyed via a probe that can be inserted vaginally or rectally.

MEDICATIONS

The cause of urinary incontinence is not necessarily something that stems from a prolapse of the vagina, uterus, bladder, or rectum. Certain medications, especially those used to treat high blood pressure (such as diuretics) and antihistamines, may cause incontinence. Adjustment in medication types and schedules may be enough to overcome incontinence. Similarly, certain medications can be somewhat effective in relaxing overactive bladder muscles or in adding muscle tone to the urethra. Specific drug therapies need to be discussed with your physician, but one regimen that would serve a multitude of purposes is estrogen replacement therapy (ERT). Estrogen via the oral or topical route can help to restore weakened support structures in a postmenopausal woman. (See Chapter 9 for more details about ERT.)

* * *

Prolapse of the pelvic structures is harmless most of the time. But this does not minimize the severe discomfort it can cause, nor does it compensate for the lifestyle changes it may impose. For example, a vaginal or uterine prolapse may interfere with sexual satisfaction, the ability to enjoy vigorous sports, or other aspects of an active life. It can cause bowel or bladder problems and even the formation of ulcers on the exposed portions of the cervix and uterus.

You may decide to undergo surgery to ameliorate some of these symptoms. Hysterectomy may be required in extreme cases. This repair can often be accomplished without hysterectomy. You may also opt for less radical solutions such as pelvic floor exercises, estrogen creams, or pessaries. In any case, this is a decision that can safely be left to *you* depending on how you feel. The gynecologist should not attempt to impose a hysterectomy, a less invasive vaginal repair, or a sacrospinous fixation on anyone whose symptoms are minimal or nonexistent.

A 1995 bulletin published by the American College of Obstetricians and Gynecologists outlined the following "surgical principles" as a guide for physicians (and patients) contemplating an operation to correct urinary incontinence:

- Surgical procedures for urinary incontinence may provide a chance for cure but are associated with more potential complications than nonsurgical approaches. Thus, operative procedures should be reserved for women who decline or do not improve following conservative therapies and, ideally, for women who have completed childbearing.

- Defects in pelvic support should be identified preoperatively, and the surgical procedure should be designed to correct current pelvic support defects as well as to prevent anatomic alterations that could cause pelvic organ prolapse postoperatively.

- There is no evidence to indicate that removal of a normal, well-supported uterus will improve the cure rate for operations designed to correct stress incontinence . . . hysterectomy generally should be reserved for gynecologic indications alone.

- Paradoxically, patients with severe pelvic organ prolapse may be continent due to the obstructive or compressive effects or both of the prolapse on the urethra. Preoperative assessment of these women should include a stress test with the prolapse reduced (the doctor can use his or her hand or an instrument to exert temporary pressure on the prolapse and hold it in place as if it were fixed) to determine if additional surgical support of the urethrovesical junction should be performed at the time of the prolapse surgery (to assure that a woman who was continent does not become incontinent after having her prolapse surgically corrected).

Thus, it's prudent to consider your options carefully and give nonsurgical techniques a fair trial before agreeing to surgery—especially hysterectomy.

If surgery is the best option, remember that it is unlikely that you would ever have just a single pelvic abnormality, such as a cystocele, without having accompanying tearing of other portions of the pelvic diaphragm. Therefore, your physician must be aware of problems with the rectal sling, the uterine sling, and the bladder sling. Remember that the rectum, bladder, and uterus are all sheathed by connective tissue, muscles, blood vessels, and nerves that suspend and support them. When these tissues have been torn, repair must take into account the fact that there are multiple tissue injuries. Because these structures have been weakened and stretched, the surgeon often faces a significant challenge to provide an adequate repair. To adequately repair these tissues, it is important that they be made pliable; therefore, hormone replacement therapy is critical for menopausal women whose tissues have lost strength and elasticity.

8

WHEN HYSTERECTOMY
IS UNAVOIDABLE

There is no success without hardship.
—SOPHOCLES

We have spent considerable time discussing the reasons to avoid hysterectomy as well as the latest alternative treatments available; however, we have also seen that there are still occasions when hysterectomy is the best and perhaps the only choice. This chapter addresses three questions of vital importance to those who are faced with inevitable hysterectomy:

1. What type of hysterectomy should I have?
2. Should I keep my ovaries?
3. Is hormone replacement therapy after hysterectomy in my best interest?

UNDERSTANDING
THE HYSTERECTOMY PROCEDURE—
CONVENTIONAL APPROACHES

The hysterectomy procedure has many variants, and it's important to define and clarify each. If your gynecologist recommends a hysterectomy, be sure that you understand exactly what he or she means by this and exactly how extensive the surgery will be. In addition, you'll want to know by what route the uterus will be removed and if the ovaries are to remain intact. Conventional hysterectomies are either abdominal or vaginal—in the latter case, all incisions are internal. Thee are different indications for these two routes, and both have advantages and disadvantages. Let's begin with a summary of the various types of hysterectomies, both abdominal and vaginal. (It may be helpful to refer to the diagrams shown in Figure 8.1.)

• *Partial or Subtotal Hysterectomy.* The entire body of the uterus is removed, but the cervix is left intact.

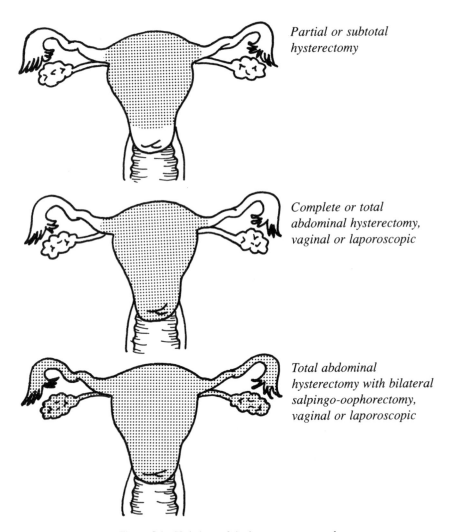

*Partial or subtotal
hysterectomy*

*Complete or total
abdominal hysterectomy,
vaginal or laporoscopic*

*Total abdominal
hysterectomy with bilateral
salpingo-oophorectomy,
vaginal or laporoscopic*

Figure 8.1 Variations of the hysterectomy procedure.

- *Complete or Total Abdominal Hysterectomy (TAH)*. The entire uterus, including the cervix, is removed, but all other pelvic structures remain.
- *Total Abdominal Hysterectomy with Bilateral Salpingo-Oophorectomy (TAH-BSO)*. Both ovaries and fallopian tubes are removed along with the uterus.
- *Radical Hysterectomy*. This operation is generally reserved for cancerous conditions of the cervix and involves removal of the uterus, ovaries, fallopian tubes, the upper portions of the vagina, and the pelvic lymph nodes.
- *The Vaginal Hysterectomy*. This operation involves making an incision in the upper portion of the vagina and removing the uterus through it. In general, only the uterus and cervix are excised in this manner, although it is technically possible for an experienced surgeon to also remove the ovaries via this route.

CHOOSING THE VAGINAL VERSUS THE ABDOMINAL APPROACH

In some cases, either a vaginal or an abdominal hysterectomy may be performed to accomplish the same goal. It's important to be familiar with the pros and cons of each approach so that you can discuss them with your surgeon.

Abdominal hysterectomies are the tried-and-true approach. An incision may be made longitudinally or crosswise—the latter is generally lower in the abdomen, perhaps below the bikini line. When extensive exploration of the abdomen is needed (as in ovarian cancer) and/or when the lymph nodes need to be removed, abdominal hysterectomy is necessary because it allows the surgeon thorough access to the pelvic cavity. For instance, if a woman has cancer or if she and her physician feel hysterectomy is absolutely necessary in a case of severe, recurrent pelvic inflammatory disease or large fibroids causing significant pelvic pain, surgery should be performed abdominally. In any case of massive pelvic adhesions or other severe pelvic pathology, the abdominal approach is necessary. In these cases, the vaginal approach is limiting and ill-advised. The highly skilled surgeon can use the laparoscopic approach to remove pelvic adhesions and treat diseased tissues within the pelvic cavity. Unfortunately, the operation itself, the hospital stay, and the recovery period are generally longer.

If your doctor tells you that he or she can "get your uterus out in thirty minutes," you should seriously consider why it is being removed in the first place. Vaginal hysterectomies are indeed quicker operations, but they require a great deal of skill. This is because there is greater potential to damage the bladder and rectum, and the operation must be performed without the benefit of a view of the abdominal cavity. Vaginal hysterectomies have limitations; for example, for a very large uterus, severe endometriosis, or other types of pelvic scar tissue, the vaginal approach is difficult and dangerous, if not impossible.

In generally, vaginal hysterectomies are best performed for a prolapsed uterus (see Chapter 7). However, sometimes vaginal hysterectomies are also done to eradicate a small fibroid or to correct recurrent uterine bleeding. A vaginal hysterectomy that is suggested for these two reasons alone can probably be avoided by using the methods we have already discussed (such as endometrial ablation). The "thirty-minute" vaginal hysterectomies that doctors boast of performing are often procedures that don't have to be done in the first place!

On the positive side of vaginal hysterectomy, it leaves no visible scar (nor is there likely to be adhesion formation) and healing will be rapid.

LAPAROSCOPIC APPROACHES TO HYSTERECTOMY

The laparoscope was introduced into gynecology about thirty years ago as a diagnostic tool. Since the first edition of this book, laparoscopic surgery as a means of treatment as well as diagnosis has really taken off, so that just about any procedure that was traditionally performed via open abdominal surgery is now being performed via the laparoscope. This is a case of caveat emptor—let the buyer (or patient) beware. It is imperative that you understand the laparoscopic procedure that is being performed, and that you engage a surgeon with extensive training and experience in these procedures, because they require more skill and different operative techniques than those learned by doctors during traditional training.

In a 1992 editorial published in the journal *Obstetrics and Gynecology*, Dr. Roy M. Pitkin raises concerns about operative laparoscopy being performed in a frenzy of popularity fueled by doctors, patients, and the media when it might not always be the best option for the patient. Questioning whether it is a "surgical advance or a technical gimmick," Dr. Pitkin poses several questions women should consider when discussing their chosen method of hysterectomy with their surgeon:

• *How does one separate technical feasibility from therapeutic appropriateness, the matter of how easily or safely or cheaply something can be done from the question of whether it should be done?* In other words, returning to the overriding theme of this book, do you even need a hysterectomy? Just because a doctor can offer you a relatively safe procedure with a relatively quick recovery time and a very small incision, are there other treatments that could allow you to preserve your pelvic organs?

- *What is the nature of quality assurance review when operations are performed outside a hospital and therefore outside the purview of regulatory or monitoring activities such as those required by the Joint Commission on Accreditation of Health Care Organizations?* This concern refers to procedures that might be performed in free-standing ambulatory surgical suites that might not have the same standards of practice as formal hospitals. Women should assure themselves that they are choosing a physician and a facility having proper credentials, training, and experience in operative laparoscopy, which is very different than the traditional training of OB-GYN doctors in general. This leads into Dr. Pitkin's next question.

- *How can appropriate credentialing criteria be established for procedures not taught in residency and for which no present member of the medical staff can claim experience?* This is changing in many parts of the country where laparoscopic hysterectomy is becoming more common, but it is still a very viable concern. Dr. Pitkin concludes his editorial by saying it is vital that the medical profession critically evaluate these newer surgical techniques—as you, the patient, should, too!

With these cautionary words in place, let us pose two more questions: How are these laparoscopic techniques performed, and how do they compare to the traditional surgical approaches? In general, laparoscopic hysterectomy is meant to take the place of abdominal, not vaginal, procedures. Almost every study conducted comparing laparoscopic techniques to traditional vaginal and open abdominal techniques found that when vaginal hysterectomy could be performed appropriately, it was the cheapest, safest, quickest, and simplest method. In other words, the laparoscope can be used in some cases to convert abdominal hysterectomy into vaginal hysterectomy, but pure laparoscopic hysterectomy should not be used as a substitute for traditional vaginal hysterectomy.

The general term "laparoscopic hysterectomy" is confusing in that it can be applied to at least three different categories of procedures: (a) diagnostic laparoscopy followed by standard vaginal hysterectomy, (2) standard laparoscopic hysterectomy, and (3) laparoscopically assisted vaginal hysterectomy.

1. Diagnostic Laparoscopy
Followed by Vaginal Hysterectomy

In this procedure, the surgeon first inserts the laparoscope to view the pelvic organs as a precursor to vaginal hysterectomy. He or she can then be assured that no condition exists that would make the vaginal approach unwise. For example, if the surgeon discovered endometriosis was present, a vaginal hysterectomy would not necessarily solve that patient's problem.

2. Standard Laparoscopic
Hysterectomy (LH)

In pure laparoscopic hysterectomy, the entire operation is performed laparoscopically, including dissection of the uterine blood vessels and removal of the uterus, ovaries, and fallopian tubes, where indicated. Vaginal hysterectomy is not appropriate for the patient who has a very large uterus, extensive endometriosis or other scar tissue, ovarian or fallopian tube disease, and/or a very long and narrow vagina. She may have a laparoscopic hysterectomy instead of open abdominal hysterectomy. Again, it must be emphasized that this procedure is technically very difficult, and a woman contemplating this type of surgery should assure herself that she is in the hands of a skilled and experienced surgeon. This operation should be performed only when your doctor considers vaginal removal of the uterus and/or other pelvic organs to be too risky or too difficult.

3. Laparoscopically Assisted Vaginal
Hysterectomy (LAVH)

This procedure blends vaginal and abdominal approaches. With the aid of the laparoscope, portions of the procedure are completed from above while the remainder (usually including the cutting away of the uterine blood vessels) is completed vaginally. This is the most common variant of laparoscopic hysterectomy performed. The beauty of the laparoscopically assisted vaginal hysterectomy is that it allows the surgeon to complete most hysterectomies that otherwise might have to be done abdominally. Pelvic adhesions, endometriosis, and ovarian cysts normally mandate that a procedure be done abdominally because of the difficulty in viewing and reaching tissues that are imbedded and bound down from vaginal approach. The ability to do this laparoscopically allows the surgeon to complete the intra-abdominal part laparoscopically and then remove the uterus through the vagina.

Pros and Cons of Laparoscopic
Versus Traditional Hysterectomy

Gynecologists continue to debate whether laparoscopic hysterectomy has anything to offer over traditional methods—whether an abdominal procedure through a 6-inch incision that can be accomplished in an hour with minimal blood loss is preferred over a two- to three-hour laparoscopic procedure. It boils down to the surgeon's skill and experience as well as the patient's need for minimized disability. I recently performed a supracervical laparoscopic hysterectomy on a woman with a very large uterus—comparable to the size of a six-month pregnancy. This turned out to be a major case that took four hours and subsequently required that the woman receive two units of blood. After the case, I questioned whether I had done the right procedure for this patient. She left the hospital in forty-eight hours, and she came to see me one week after surgery—effusive in her praise and very pleased with her results. This woman particularly desired to avoid an abdominal hysterectomy because she is a single working mother and could not take the time for a prolonged recovery, which would have been necessary from abdominal surgery. Therefore, doctors must consider what is important to the patient.

In today's climate of wanting to save on costs, to lessen the discomfort and complications, and to have women back to their daily routines as quickly, safely, and efficiently as possible, laparoscopic hysterectomy is certainly appropriate in certain cases. Most doctors would agree that a standard vaginal hysterectomy—when indicated and necessary—is the best method of all. However, only 28 percent of hysterectomies nationwide are performed vaginally. Over 70 percent are still done via the open abdominal route. Abdominal hysterectomies have the highest rates of complications with the longest postoperative hospital stays (about six days) and the lengthiest overall recovery times (at least six weeks). Therefore, LAVH, a technique of laparoscopic dissection coupled with vaginal removal of the uterus and other pelvic organs, was developed to "convert" an abdominal hysterectomy into a vaginal hysterectomy.

LH and LAVH are often criticized for being costlier and longer procedures. The higher costs stem from extended operating room time and the use of video monitors and expensive disposable laparoscopic instruments. However, advocates of these surgeries point to the fact that as surgeons become more experienced and rely more on reusable as opposed to disposable instruments, costs and operating time goes down. Supporters also say that women who undergo LH are in the hospital only a day or two; thus the cost of keeping someone in the hospital and its associated skilled nursing care is lower. In addition, LH and LAVH have a complication rate that is lower than traditional abdominal hysterectomy (16 percent versus 20 percent; but vaginal hysterectomy rate is lowest at 12 percent). Another tremendous advantage of LAVH is that it allows the physician to look inside the abdomen at the conclusion of the procedure to make sure that all bleeding points have been sealed and coagulated. I can recall a number of times when I thought that all the tissues were dry and the procedure was completed, but when I took a final look through the laparoscope, I found some oozing and bleeding points. This final look has saved my patients a number of complications.

Women generally prefer the laparoscopic approach because it results in less pain and a much smaller scar than does open abdominal surgery. It even offers some advantages over standard vaginal hysterectomy: Hospital stays are still shorter by a couple of days, it is easier to control bleeding, and easier to inspect and remove the ovaries and fallopian tubes.

Dr. Camran Nezhat and his colleagues may have put it best in a 1994 issue of *Obstetrics and Gynecology*. Reporting their analysis of the various operative techniques of hysterectomies, they said:

> Patients strongly favor laparoscopy-assisted vaginal hysterectomy because of the smaller incision, diminished postoperative pain, shorter hospital stay, and quicker return to normal activity. Because modern medicine values patient comfort and pain reduction, converting a laparotomy [open abdominal surgery] to a minimal access procedure has undeniable benefits. In the final analysis, it may be difficult to place a monetary amount on the decreased pain and discomfort achieved by performing laparoscopy-assisted vaginal hysterectomy instead of abdominal hysterectomy.

Consider also the cautionary words of Dr. John Steege, writing in the *American Journal of Obstetrics and Gynecology*:

> ... [D]id the availability and alleged advantages of laparoscopically-assisted vaginal hysterectomy prompt more women to seek out surgery they would otherwise have avoided? Did the physicians' enthusiasm for the alleged benefits of the procedure translate into easier acceptance of surgery? ... I stand with those who believe that the laparoscopically-assisted vaginal hysterectomy, properly used in appropriately selected cases, is a significant improvement in our surgical methods. . . . But the true challenge remains: using the procedure in a spirit of caution rather than competition, allowing it to take its proper place as a refinement, rather than an unneeded expansion, of health care for women.

SPEEDING YOUR RECOVERY

In either case, it's important to have a frank discussion with your physician regarding what to expect during the recovery period. Immediately after the surgery, and no matter how uncomfortable you may feel, you should try to walk with assistance. Remaining stationary retards circulation and increases your risk of developing thrombophlebitis (blood clots) in your legs. In addition, you should follow the coughing and deep breathing instructions that you will no doubt be taught by a nurse.

Both of these steps decrease the likelihood of developing pneumonia after the surgery. (Lying immobile in bed allows fluid to accumulate in the lungs. This serves as a perfect incubating medium for bacteria, and hence pneumonia may result.)

Because of the economics of health care, patients are being discharged from hospitals much sooner postoperatively than in the past. You must be your own advocate in scheduling your discharge. If you feel weak, dizzy, nauseated, and are scheduled for discharge on the day of surgery or the day after, be sure to have the nurse note your symptoms fully and then notify the nursing staff that you are not able to go home. Insurance companies will allow extended stays if there is documented evidence of a requirement for a longer hospitalization. It serves no useful purpose to drag yourself home before you are well enough.

It's also important to recognize that being sent home doesn't mean you are ready to resume your former role of superwoman. Remember, you may need to be on pain medications, and these can affect your judgment. Arrange for someone to take care of you (and any young children) for as long as possible. Avoid lifting heavy loads, moving large objects, doing major housework, and driving for as long as your doctor tells you is necessary. Again, discuss with your doctor when you can resume working, having sex, douching, and participating in very active sports. Expect that it may be two or more months before you can again be fully functional. Be sure to contact your physician if you develop a fever, worsening pain, significant bleeding, or discharge from the wound.

BEING YOUR OWN ADVOCATE— KEEPING YOUR OVARIES

One should never forget that ovarian cancer is a very serious disease, difficult to detect, difficult to manage, and ultimately deadly for one in every hundred women. No doubt this has prompted surgeons to remove innumerable ovaries over the years. However, nymphomania was once considered a serious disease, and zealous surgeons used to cavalierly remove the ovaries of women who in their opinion suffered from that condition.

According to the American College of Obstetricians and Gynecologists, an estimated seven hundred prophylactic oophorectomies would be required to prevent a single case of ovarian cancer! And, in light of the sometimes dramatic and debilitating effects associated with "instant menopause" (see Chapter 9), it is in the best interest of every woman and her doctor to carefully weigh the pros and cons of oophorectomy. For example, a premenopausal woman undergoing hysterectomy and oophorectomy has three times the risk of developing coronary artery disease and is thus much more likely to die of a heart condition than from any form of cancer, ovarian or otherwise.

Even more troubling are reports in the scientific literature of women developing cancer identical to ovarian cancer years after bilateral oophorectomy! Doctors still don't understand this phenomenon, although it may be related to ovarian cancer being able to develop in abdominal tissue that was a precursor to ovary formation in the embryo. Thus, removing your ovaries is not a 100 percent guarantee that you will never develop ovarian cancer.

If you are to have your ovaries removed, you should probably undergo estrogen replacement therapy (ERT) to minimize the side effects discussed in Chapter 9, especially osteoporosis and cardiovascular disease. Yet, as we shall see, this is a major decision with some disadvantages and some risks. Furthermore, not every woman is willing or able to take hormonal supplements for what may be the rest of her life. Finally, ERT does not solve all of the potential and troublesome side effects (i.e., skin changes and decreased sexual desire), because it cannot substitute for what nature provides. Consider this statement by the American College of Obstetricians and Gynecologists:

> Hormonal replacement with estrogen and a progestogen [progesterone] is not physiologic. In premenopausal women who have undergone oophorectomy, gonadotrophin [sex hormone] levels do not return to premenopausal levels following estrogen-progestogen therapy, indicating that feedback control on the hypothalamic-pituitary axis [nervous system] is incompletely mimicked by these two exogenous hormones.

Some surgeons try to convince women to have their ovaries removed at the time of hysterectomy to prevent them from needing another operation in the future. For most women, another operation will never be necessary. The incidence of repeat operations for removal of residual ovaries is less than 5 percent. Looked at from another angle, of all the women with ovarian cancer, few have had a prior hysterectomy. (Estimates vary widely, from fewer than 1 percent to no more than 14 percent.)

You should consider certain criteria when deciding whether to preserve your ovaries. Your age is important. Ovarian cancer is extremely rare before age forty, and menopause is not likely to occur for a number of years. Therefore, don't let anyone talk you into a prophylactic oophorectomy before your fortieth birthday. It may, however, be reasonable to have an oophorectomy after age fifty, and I may advise a woman to do so. When it's not a life-or-death decision, but more a consideration of how a woman may feel faced with the loss of her ovaries (she is now castrated), I firmly believe that it is the role of the gynecologist to advise, inform, and guide her in her decision—not to make the decision for her. It is she who is going to have to live with the consequences and with her feelings afterward; therefore, it is she who must make the ultimate choice after informed and thoughtful consideration.

Other factors besides age may tip the balance either in favor of or against this procedure. Oophorectomy may make sense depending on your personal or family medical history. For example, if you have had ovarian cysts or endometriosis, you may find that pain recurs or persists after your hysterectomy, necessitating oophorectomy. If you have had breast, endometrial, or colon cancer, you are at increased risk for ovarian cancer and should consider prophylactic oophorectomy. Likewise, having close relatives with breast or ovarian cancer increases your risk. Conversely, situations that have allowed the ovary to rest for a while, such as having had children or having taken birth control pills (even for as short a time as three months), statistically decrease ovarian cancer risk and should be taken into consideration.

All in all, it is a complex decision that requires you to weigh your risks against your willingness to weather the menopausal storm, which can be expected to be more severe when induced surgically.

SHOULD YOU KEEP YOUR CERVIX?

The topic of conservation of the cervix during hysterectomy is controversial. Fifty years ago, most hysterectomies were subtotal, meaning that the cervix was left intact; later, total hysterectomy was favored because of the fear of cervical cancer. Since the Pap smear has come into such widespread use since the 1950s, we can now look more critically at the role of the cervix. The cervix supports the lower genital diaphragm and also serves as a protective barrier as well as a vital passage. The cervix is also believed to play a role in female sexual response, including lubrication.

Many physicians now advocate cervical conservation during abdominal hysterectomy. The problem is that it is very difficult to preserve the cervix during a vaginal or a laparoscopic hysterectomy. In these procedures, the cervical attachments are removed before the main body of the uterus is extracted. I don't have a good answer to this dilemma; however, I want to make you aware of the issue so that you can discuss it with your surgeon. Saving the cervix is not necessarily crucial for all women, but it is a decision you should have a role in making along with your doctor. Supracervical hysterectomy (cervical conservation) has both benefits and drawbacks, so you need to hear the pros and cons in your particular case from your physician before a method of surgery is decided upon.

HORMONE REPLACEMENT— CONSIDER IT CAREFULLY

The development of hormone supplements to curb the deleterious effects of menopause has proven to be a tremendous advance in women's health care. They are relatively safe (not seeming to share some of the worrisome side effects of their distant relative, birth control pills). They are now conveniently available as creams, suppositories, and transdermal patches as well as the traditional tablets and injections. (*Note:* The patches are placed on the skin, and the medication slowly releases in a controlled dosage over several days. The hormones seem to bypass the liver when they are being processed by the body, and therefore may have fewer side effects. For this reason they may not be as effective for all postmenopausal indications.) However, despite safety, efficacy, and improved convenience, ERT remains controversial (see Table 8.1).

Endometrial Cancer Risk

In the mid-1970s, two highly regarded studies published in the *New England Journal of Medicine* cited a substantially increased risk of endometrial cancer associated with estrogen use. To make matters worse, these frightening results were confirmed in the numerous investigations that followed, sometimes revealing as much as an eightfold increase in risk—a risk that did not go away even if a woman stopped taking estrogen. In short order, the fountain of youth had turned into a dance with death. Doctors stopped prescribing estrogen, and women stopped taking it.

Table 8.1   Hormone Replacement Therapy: Should You or Shouldn't You?

Estrogen

Advantages

Relieves hot flashes and flushes.
May help with bladder dysfunction and discomforts.
Reverses aging effects on vagina.
Prevents osteoporosis.
May prevent heart disease by altering cholesterol.
May help with insomnia, especially if due to nocturnal flushes.

Disadvantages

May have unpleasant side effects, such as breast tenderness, weight gain, nausea, headaches.
May cause high blood pressure (dose related).
If taken without progesterone, carries increased risk of endometrial cancer.
May increase risk of gallbladder disease.

Progesterone

Advantages

May help with emotional state, depending on underlying causes and other life events.
May help sex life, especially if problems are related to vaginal discomforts.
Seems to negate endometrial cancer risk for women on ERT.
May prevent breast cancer; extremely controversial.

Disadvantages

May increase chance of breast cancer; extremely controversial.
May cause vaginal bleeding, weight gain or increased appetite, mood swings, breast tenderness, or acne (temporary phenomena).
May eliminate benefits of ERT on the heart due to increase in LDL cholesterol.

Testosterone

Advantages

Generally increases libido.*
May help reduce hot flashes.

Disadvantages

May cause masculinizing side effects, such as growth of facial hair, lowering of vocal register, and acne.

*Unlike estrogen, which seems to aid in sexual dysfunction mainly by increasing vaginal lubrication and preventing atrophic vaginitis, testosterone seems to increase sexual arousal and orgasms.

In subsequent years, further work determined that so-called unopposed estrogen was at the root of the danger. This was because constant exposure of the uterus to estrogen, as in the case of naturally occurring hormonal imbalance and dysfunctional uterine bleeding, leads to endometrial hyperplasia. Hyperplasia may lead to cancer.

It was determined that if, as in the premenopausal state, a woman was given progesterone in addition to estrogen, this abnormal buildup of the uterine lining would be circumvented. Today, estrogen replacement therapy has regained its good name, but it is highly recommended that it be cycled with a progesterone in women who still have their uterus.

Of course, progesterone is not without its price. Depending on the type of progesterone you take, the cardioprotective effects of estrogen may be somewhat negated. Specifically, progesterone increases LDL cholesterol. Therefore, it's important that you take a type of progesterone least likely to have this effect, and that you take it long enough to protect against cancer (at least seven to ten days each month).

Finally, be prepared for the fact that estrogen with progesterone may again make you feel as you did when you were menstruating. You may experience a return of acne, breast tenderness, mood swings, and perhaps most inconvenient of all, vaginal bleeding. Some of these side effects may be ameliorated by adjusting the dosage of the progesterone. More important, many women consider all of these side effects worthwhile to protect themselves against osteoporosis, cardiac disease, and endometrial cancer.

Breast Cancer Risk

In 1988 doctors at the Mayo Clinic very effectively summarized the available information on hormone replacement therapy and the risk of breast cancer:

> Methodologic deficiencies and inconsistencies have prevented a clear understanding of whether estrogen replacement therapy increases the risk of breast cancer. Some investigators have shown that a slight but statistically insignificant increased risk of breast cancer is associated with the oral use of estrogens. Others have concluded that estrogens do not increase the risk of breast cancer and may improve the prognosis in those in whom breast cancer does develop during estrogen therapy. In any event, the risk seems to be small and has not been found consistently. . . .

Believe it or not, this statement doesn't begin to highlight all of the confusion and controversy surrounding this particular issue. The following are some of the unanswered questions.

Is dosage and duration of therapy important? Some researchers believe that how much estrogen you take and for how long is the link to breast cancer. One large study found long-term use in moderately high doses could be linked to breast cancer, whereas short-term, low-dose therapy could not.

How important is the way in which you take the estrogen? A group of investigators in North Carolina revealed that the risk of breast cancer with oral forms was negligible, but that injectable estrogen increased the risk fourfold. However, lest you gain a false sense of security from pill use, a study of over 23,000 Swedish women published in a 1989 issue of the *New En-gland Journal of Medicine* seems to indicate that not all oral estrogens may be created equal. That is, the type of oral estrogen you take may make the difference between no risk and nearly double the risk of breast cancer. (Fortunately, the safest estrogen pills are also those most commonly prescribed in the United States. Specifically, synthetic so-called estradiol-type estrogens were implicated, whereas natural estrogens were not.)

Can progesterone safeguard against any increased risk of breast cancer? A 1986 editorial appearing in *Obstetrics and Gynecology* seemed at first to support this view, citing the evidence of two well-publicized studies by Dr. Gambrell and his colleagues. However, claiming that these investigations had "serious methodologic flaws," the editors concluded that "[c]urrent evidence does not justify the practice of adding progestin to postmenopausal estrogen therapy in an attempt to reduce the risk of breast cancer."

Do women with benign breast disease (i.e., "cystic breasts") add to their risk of developing cancer if they take ERT? Likewise, what about women who have had their ovaries removed? Again, it depends on which scientific study you believe. Some say taking ERT reduces breast cancer risk; others directly contradict them! In one study of Australian women, breast cancer risk reduction in both of these areas was dramatic: 40 percent for women with benign breast disease; 70 percent for women with bilateral oophorectomy. In another study, by British physicians, "[The] most consistently identified [risk factor for breast cancer] has been a history of benign breast disease." Furthermore, these same doctors found that "[a]lthough hormone use was not associated with any substantial overall risk, there was some hazard suggested among women who have received hormones following bilateral oophorectomy."

Is it advisable to commence ERT if there is a family history of breast cancer? Dr. Phyllis Wingo and her colleagues (*Journal of the American Medical Association*, 1987) found a "twofold increased risk" if women had a close relative who had breast cancer.

The most frustrating aspect to this, of course, is that neither doctors nor patients receive concrete and consistent information. Clearly, additional work needs to be done. We need to discover whether women will exhibit the increased incidence of breast cancer found when laboratory animals are given ERT. We must resolve whether estrogen supplementation will increase breast cancer risk in the same manner as do conditions that naturally increase estrogen exposure, such as obesity, infrequent or late pregnancies, and hormonal imbalance. Finally, we must face the fact that all of the data—pro and con—must be tempered by time; that is, cancer often takes many years to show itself. For example, workers exposed to asbestos as young men did not begin to reveal exorbitant rates of lung cancer for twenty to thirty years.

For now, the best we can do is act with caution. It's probably not a good idea to take ERT if you already have a significant risk factor for breast cancer. In addition, special attention should be devoted to regular, thorough breast self-examinations and to having mammograms according to the recommended guidelines for women over age thirty-five. This advice applies whether or not you ultimately decide to take estrogen.

Incidentally, cervical cancer and ovarian cancer do not appear to be affected by hormone replacement therapy.

Other Risks

Many of the official contraindications to ERT are based on some of the problems that have been known to develop when women have been on birth control pills. As already mentioned, oral contraceptives differ fundamentally in type and dosage from postmenopausal hormone supplements. Nevertheless, until researchers know more, it is best to err on the safe side. Because estrogen is processed by the liver, ERT is not advised for women with either liver or gallbladder disease. In addition, because it may affect blood clotting, estrogen should be avoided if you have had a blood clot form in your leg (phlebitis) or if one has blocked off the blood supply to your heart or brain, resulting respectively in either a heart attack or a stroke. In order to avoid any contribution to arteriosclerotic heart disease, have your blood pressure and cholesterol checked before embarking on ERT. Finally, certain preexisting medical conditions (e.g., migraine headaches, endometriosis, and fibroids) may worsen with ERT and thus require careful watching.

Benefits of Estrogen Replacement

I always want to hear the bad news first, then you can tell me the good news. You have heard the bad news, or potential risks, of ERT. The good news is that most doctors today would agree that overall, ERT is a good idea for postmenopausal women for several reasons: It is available in a variety of forms that make it both safe and convenient to take. It can temper the annoying side effects of menopause, such as hot flushes, vaginal dryness, and decreased libido. In addition, and perhaps more essential, it can help women to avoid the serious toll that cardiac disease and osteoporosis can take once natural estrogen levels decline. (For more information about the aftermath of hysterectomy and the effects of menopause, see Chapter 9.)

* * *

To minimize the damage that may be done when hysterectomy cannot be avoided, it's important to consider several factors including whether you can choose the type of hysterectomy you have, and whether you can safely preserve your ovaries to avoid making an undesirable situation worse. (See the box on page 154.)

If you have this surgery, you should certainly consider the relative advantages and disadvantages of hormonal replacement therapy in your case. No set rules and regulations apply. On the positive side, as discussed at length in Chapter 9, ERT can help to reverse such unpleasant side effects as hot flushes, atrophic vaginitis, bladder discomfort, and perhaps even depression and sexual difficulties. More important, it will most likely impact on your risk for osteoporosis and arteriosclerosis—both deadly diseases.

However, you may be exposing yourself to a greater risk of breast cancer and possibly other serious medical conditions, such as thrombophlebitis. (Remember, the incidence of thrombophlebitis is a lot lower with ERT than with oral contraceptives.) Furthermore, ERT requires years of compliance with taking medications that may cause unpleasant side effects. This is an inconvenience many women find unacceptable.

If you decide to take hormonal replacement, insist on the lowest effective dose, and discuss with the doctor whether less invasive routes, such as transdermal patches, will be effective in accomplishing your goal. You must be diligent when it comes to following through with screening tests to monitor your health while on ERT. These include regular blood pressure readings, blood tests for cholesterol levels, breast and pelvic exams (including mammograms, Pap smears, and periodic endometrial biopsies, as needed). Endometrial biopsies are important because they will assure you and your physician that hyperplasia is not present. Sometimes an endovaginal ultrasound scan can replace the more uncomfortable endometrial biopsy procedure. An ultrasound will help the doctor to determine if the lining of the uterus is normal or thickened; if it is thickened, an endometrial biopsy needs to be performed.

The rewards of hormone replacement therapy may be a longer, more productive life! Consider this statement by Drs. Hillner, Hollenberg, and Pauker, which was published in the *American Journal of Medicine* in 1986:

Questions to Ask if Your Doctor Recommends a Hysterectomy

WHO is this doctor? Is he or she someone you know and trust? Does he or she have a good reputation in the community, and are his or her credentials beyond reproach? Even so, get a second— even a third—opinion before consenting to surgery.

WHAT does the doctor intend to take out? Believe it or not, in talking to women who have had hysterectomies, some do not know exactly what was removed! Remember all the variations and per- mutations of hysterectomy, and make sure you understand clearly if only your uterus is to be removed. If so, is it your entire uterus or will the cervix be left behind? Will the ovaries, fallopian tubes, lymph nodes, portions of the vagina, appendix, or other tissues also be taken out? If so, why? If not, why not? *Make sure that you are es- pecially clear about and comfortable with the discussion concerning removal of your ovaries. Try to have a say in the matter when there is a choice, and consider all the pros and cons in your case.*

WHEN does the surgery need to be done? Postpone schedul- ing the operation if it is not clearly an emergency. (Most of the time, it isn't.) Allow yourself time to seek other opinions, to care- fully consider what the loss of your uterus will mean to you and your partner, and to adjust to the idea if you elect to proceed with hysterectomy. Women who did this had significantly fewer psycho- logical problems afterward than those who rushed ahead.

WHERE will the incision be made? Do you have a choice of vaginal versus abdominal hysterectomy? How about laparoscopic options? For extensive pelvic disease, you want to campaign for an abdominal procedure, whereas vaginal hysterectomies are preferred for prolapse. *(If a vaginal hysterectomy is not being performed for a prolapse, chances are it doesn't have to be done at all.)* If a sur- geon is comfortable with abdominal hysterectomies, don't try to talk him or her into doing a vaginal one or vice versa. If a doctor is unfamiliar with laparoscopic techniques, don't try to get him or her to attempt a laparoscopic procedure. Instead, find a doctor who is an expert at the procedure you desire.

WHY do you need this hysterectomy? Remember that obviously the best "damage control" for hysterectomies is avoiding them! Now that you have read this book, you know that the so-called indica- tions for hysterectomies do not mean that they are truly "necessary." There may be alternative treatments, and there may be time to "watch and wait." *Don't let anyone—not even a renowned physi- cian with a lot of impressive degrees and credentials—talk you into a hysterectomy if you feel uncomfortable with the idea. Carefully consider the options. Remember, what is done cannot be undone!*

[E]strogen therapy provides a significant gain in quality-adjusted life expectancy. In considering the efficacy of any drug, all the benefits of the drug as well as all its risks must be included. If the beneficial effect of estrogens on cardiovascular mortality is confirmed, it will overshadow all other effects. Any recommendation about postmenopausal estrogens with respect to osteoporosis that excludes their cardiovascular effects markedly underestimates the potential gains from therapy.

Dr. Elizabeth Barrett-Conner (*New England Journal of Medicine*, 1989) adds:

For the average North American woman, who will be postmenopausal for one third of her life, the benefits of estrogen seem strongly established. In addition to its unequivocal value for the relief of menopausal symptoms, the long-term use of postmenopausal estrogen can prevent osteoporosis and its debilitating or fatal consequences. The use of estrogen must also be considered in light of a possible 50 percent reduction in the risk of cardiovascular disease and the possibility of a nearly doubled risk of breast cancer. In this decade the increased risk of endometrial cancer associated with estrogen use led to the frequent addition of a progestin to estrogen-replacement therapy, which further complicates the tallying of risks and benefits.

Up to now, we've examined all of the options both for avoiding hysterectomy whenever possible, and for maintaining damage control when hysterectomy is unavoidable. In the next chapter, we will talk about what you might expect to experience in the aftermath of hysterectomy as well as how to handle the effects.

PART THREE

THE AFTERMATH—
TAKING BACK
CONTROL OF YOUR
BODY

I still hear stories every day from patients who say, "He wanted to clean me all out, so I wouldn't have to worry any more." "Clean me out" is a most disturbing expression. Does the doctor consider the uterus and ovaries dirty? Is the patient really cleaner without them?

I recently spent an hour at a teaching conference at Harvard Medical School. Problem patients were being presented for physicians' recommendations as to how they should best be treated. One patient was a 73-year-old man with prostate cancer. The urologist was extremely concerned with his therapy, as was the radiation therapist. The conversation went something like this:

Urologist: I think that a surgical approach might work, but I am really afraid that it would make him impotent.

Radiotherapist: Yes, but I'm not sure if the tumor can be well radiated because of its position. Radiation may not be a good choice for him.

Urologist: I am concerned. I wouldn't want him to lose his potency. Surgery in that area may ruin his sex life.

I almost had to pinch myself to make sure I wasn't dreaming. Here we have a patient with a spreading cancer who is 73 years old. His surgeon is carrying on and on about his sexuality. I'm not against sex, but where are the surgeons who defend women's sexuality when they are presented for castration (removal of the ovaries) in the hundreds of thousands? I have never heard so much as a peep from my surgical colleagues on their behalf.

No one ever seems to consider what the consequences might be for the woman and what it might do to her body image. I suppose if you are a man, it might seem that the loss of a uterus and ovaries is not important to a woman's sexuality. She can still have a sex life. And if her scar is well hidden, how could she ever know the difference? What they fail to realize is that women have feelings about their sexual organs, too. They may not be visible, but I still think that they are precious to us.

—PENNY WISE BUDOFF, M.D.
No More Hot Flashes and Other Good News

9

COPING WITH
THE AFTERMATH

*It is important to understand that it is normal to mourn the loss
of your reproductive capability. It is equally important to
recognize that each woman will grieve in her own way.*
—WANDA WIGFALL WILLIAMS, clinical psychologist, 1982

Since the turn of the century, remarkable advances in medicine and technology have succeeded in doubling the life expectancy of American women, who may now survive to an average age of approximately eighty years. This means that a woman can expect to spend a third of her life in the menopausal state. There are presently more than 35 million postmenopausal women in the United States for whom attitudes and approaches to menopause have important repercussions.

Is menopause a "disease" we need to "cure"? Dr. Wulf Utian argues in "The Fate of the Untreated Menopause": "As a result of my 20 years of research on menopause, I now believe that menopause may be considered an endocrinopathy." If so, then what are the symptoms, and left untreated, what will be the adverse effects? What is the best "therapy"?

Menopause is accompanied by several important physiologic changes, which not all women will experience equally. In addition, it cannot be debated that some of these changes are viewed as positive by the majority of women; that is, no more menstrual periods and no more fear of unwanted pregnancy. However, many of these changes are not positive, and they have varying degrees of serious impact on the older woman's health status.

INSTANT MENOPAUSE

For women who undergo a natural menopause, physiologic changes occur very gradually and may be nearly unnoticeable, with a slight decline in ovarian function beginning in the late thirties or early forties and extending over a period of fifteen or twenty years, until the actual cessation of

159

menses. (See Figure 9.1.) However, no woman is as acutely aware of the changes in her body as the one who has undergone an instant menopause brought on by a hysterectomy, especially when accompanied by an oophorectomy.

If the image of a woman in certain segments of our society is irreversibly tied to her reproductive capability, what does this say about her worth after menopause, and how do these attitudes impact on her psychological state? From a historical perspective, menopause has certainly been looked on in an unfavorable light. Here is a passage from an 1845 book entitled *Treatise on the Diseases of Females*: "Compelled to yield to the power of time, women now cease to exist for the species, and henceforward live only for themselves. Their features are stamped with the impress of age, and their genital organs are sealed with the signet of sterility."

This chapter will attempt to place menopause in its proper perspective—to present an objective look at the mental and physical changes you may experience as a result of menopause, especially when accelerated by pelvic surgery. It will present some of the coping strategies you may employ to help you to continue to lead a healthy, long, and active life. Key to this discussion will be the role of hormone replacement therapy, which was introduced in the last chapter.

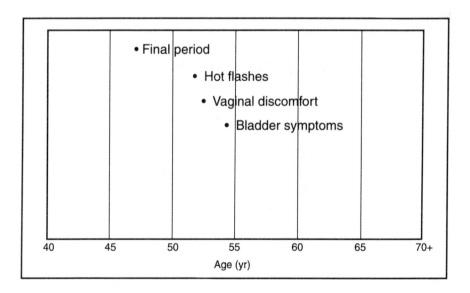

Figure 9.1 Graph of menstrual changes over time.

HOW WOMEN CHANGE
WITH THE "CHANGE OF LIFE"

Estrogens are vital organic compounds that are not the exclusive property of human women. Indeed, estrogens or receptors for estrogenlike compounds have been identified in men, lower animals, and even plants! That estrogens exert their influence throughout the human body (and not merely in the genital tract) is proven by the presence of estrogen receptors in many organs, ranging from the skin to the brain and spinal cord, colon, pancreas, liver, adrenal glands, bladder, heart, and arteries. It is no wonder, then, that with menopause and the steady decline of ovarian estrogen production, the physiologic effects are seen and felt far and wide. (See Table 9.1.)

Table 9.1   Bodily Changes with Menopause

Organ	Symptom	Helped by Estrogen Replacement Therapy?
Uterus	Shrinkage in size and decreased muscle tone; weakening of support structures predisposing to prolapse.	Yes
Ovary	Cessation of ovulation and menstruation; loss of the ability to conceive.	No
Breasts	Reduction in size; weakening of support structures causing sagging of tissue.	Yes
Bladder	Thinning of tissues; increased susceptibility to infections and prolapse due to weakened support structures; causes increased frequency of urination and stress incontinence.	Yes
Nervous system	Hot flashes/flushes; depression; sleep disturbances; sexual dysfunction.	Yes
Skin	Increased thinning and dryness with associated itching.	Maybe
Hair	Increased dryness, thinning, and loss; possible facial hair development.	Maybe
Skeleton	Decreased bone mass with resulting osteoporosis.	Yes
Heart and blood vessels	Increased risk of cardiovascular disease, mainly attributed to changes in blood cholesterol.	Yes
Vulva	Shrinkage in size and fatty tissue; more susceptible to rashes and itching.	Yes
Vagina	Increased dryness and thinning of tissues; more susceptible to vaginitis and painful intercourse.	Yes

Ironically, the earliest effects, which are the ones that produce the most noticeable symptoms (e.g., hot flashes), are not necessarily the most lasting or the most serious in the long term. In the 1960s, it was for these symptoms that estrogen replacement therapy (ERT) was touted as the "fountain of youth" that would keep women "forever feminine." A decade later, ERT fell out of favor when several research studies linked it to cancer. Today, hormone replacement therapy (HRT)—in a modified form—is again being recommended.

Frequently, menopausal symptoms may be ameliorated—even eliminated—by hormone replacement therapy, which is now safer and more convenient than ever. Prempro is a combination pill that includes estrogen and progesterone in one formulation. Unlike the cycled ERT regimens of the past (where you would take several weeks of estrogen followed by a week of progesterone), Prempro can be taken daily to avoid, for most women, the return to periodic vaginal bleeding, which once served as a major obstacle. Its most frequently cited side effect is breast discomfort. To ameliorate this effect, some women take cycled Prempro. The good news is that even when cycled for twenty-five days out of the month with one week off the medication, at least half of all women will stop bleeding after about six months of therapy. Any woman who has breakthrough bleeding (vaginal bleeding during the time when she is taking active hormonal medication) should let her doctor know immediately, because up to 80 percent of these women have some abnormality of the uterus. Use of HRT should be seriously considered by all women who have no major contraindications to it in order to safeguard against osteoporosis and heart disease—two enemies of the mature woman. More will be said about this later in the chapter. For now, let's look at the early effects of estrogen depletion.

Hot Flashes and Flushes

These are the earliest and most commonly experienced effects of menopause. Experts estimate that as many as 75 to 85 percent of women undergoing menopause (naturally or via oophorectomy) will experience hot flashes and flushes for at least a year, with up to 50 percent of women saying that they lasted for five to ten years. Although not seeming to be a serious problem to those fortunate enough to be spared the effects, we know from the great numbers of women who seek medical attention for this problem that hot flashes and flushes may substantially interfere with the quality of life during both waking and sleeping hours. Most severely affected are those who experience "instant menopause," either via surgery or radiation.

A hot flash is the subjective premonition by the woman that she is about to experience a hot flush. Unlike flashes, hot flushes can be objectively measured: A definite change in temperature and pulse is accompanied by the temporary, but sudden and profound, stretching of the blood vessels found in the skin of the face, neck, and upper chest. This in turn causes increased blood flow to the area with profuse sweating. The underlying mechanism for these events seems to be a drop in estrogen levels that disrupts the hypothalamus—the body's "thermostat." For unknown reasons, hot flushes seem to occur most commonly during the night, often disturbing a woman's rest. She may wake frequently and sometimes have to change her nightgown or the sheets. Some doctors have even hypothesized that the psychological symptoms some women complain of during menopause, such as fatigue, insomnia, irritability, difficulty concentrating, and depression, may actually be a result of sleep deprivation secondary to hot flushes.

Numerous studies have concluded that ERT has beneficial effects on hot flashes and flushes. The American College of Obstetrics and Gynecology recently summarized these conclusions: "Estrogen therapy effectively decreases the frequency and severity of subjective symptoms as well as the objective signs of menopausal flushes. With discontinuation of therapy, the symptoms may recur; gradually reducing the dose of estrogen in this situation, however, frequently minimizes the problem."

Progesterone, testosterone, and clonidine (a blood pressure medication) have also been demonstrated to alleviate hot flushes, although not as dramatically as estrogen. Estrogen remains the treatment of choice for this problem.

Vaginal Discomfort

Over time, estrogen deficiency may also cause changes in the anatomy and physiology of your vaginal area. The skin and hair covering the external structures (vulva) become thinner. Within the vagina, changes occur in the cells that comprise its structure and in the chemicals these cells produce. The vagina becomes drier, thinner, and shorter in some cases, thus making intercourse more uncomfortable for some women. In addition, the vagina may be more easily injured and irritated. Because of chemical changes, the premenopausal milieu that maintained a natural resistance to foreign bacterial invaders is altered, causing you to be more susceptible to infections. The discharge and irritation that may result from trauma and infections related to menopause is called atrophic vaginitis. Symptoms include burning, itching, white or clear discharge, and occasionally even bleeding.

If a woman remains sexually active during the menopausal years, these effects may be minimized or prevented. The mechanics of intercourse may keep the vagina from shortening. In addition, some doctors hypothesize that steroids from the man's ejaculate may be absorbed by the woman, resulting in an effect similar to estrogen replacement therapy.

Hormone replacement therapy has been found to be effective in reversing the vaginal changes associated with menopause. One study found that symptoms of vaginitis resolved in 89 percent of women, painful intercourse in 73 percent, and vaginal itching in 68 percent. Estrogen creams applied directly to the vagina are as effective as taking pills, and they may be more appealing to some women. You may also benefit from the use of water-based lubricants during intercourse to ease the discomfort and potential damage from the friction against fragile vaginal tissues.

Bladder Symptoms

The cells of the bladder and urethra (the structure leading from the bladder that allows the passage of urine from the body) are similar to the vagina in their response to declining levels of estrogen. There may be irritation and increased susceptibility to infections because of thinning of these tissues. Some women also develop difficulties with incontinence when estrogen depletion causes them to lose muscle tone in their pelvic floor. As discussed in Chapter 7, the pelvic floor may be stretched during childbirth and the bladder may prolapse into the vagina causing women to leak urine when they strain, cough, or laugh. Other estrogen-related changes affect the regulation of urine flow so that urine may remain in the bladder for prolonged periods, again predisposing a woman to infections. HRT is effective in reversing many of the bladder symptoms of menopause and may help women to avoid hysterectomy from these causes.

The Skin

Several years ago, a television commercial advertising a dishwashing product displayed a mother's and daughter's hands side by side. You weren't supposed to be able to tell the difference between these two women's ages until the camera panned to their faces. Thus far, science has been unable to prove that dishwashing liquid has any beneficial effect on slowing the effects of aging on skin! The skin contains estrogen receptors and is believed to be a major target of menopausal changes. It's also the most exposed organ of the body and subject to the greatest environmental influences. Therefore, it's difficult to determine whether the thinning, drying, and wrinkling result from the cumulative effects of many years of daily wear and tear—all of those suntanning sessions, for example—or from estrogen depletion. It's likely that both contribute to the overall aging of a woman's skin. Unfortunately, hormone replacement has not been established to be any more effective than dishwashing liquid in reversing these symptoms. Here's what doctors at the Mayo Clinic have to say about HRT for skin changes: "Estrogen is not a panacea for aging, and no available data prove that estrogen therapy confers cosmetic benefits." The American College of Obstetrics and Gynecology adds, "The effects of estrogen replacement therapy on the skin . . . have not been clearly established. Until a beneficial cosmetic effect is demonstrated, the use of estrogen for this purpose cannot be recommended."

While I personally don't believe that estrogen can restore wrinkled skin, I do believe that ERT begun early in menopause will prevent or retard skin breakdown. Sun exposure is the primary cause of skin damage. We all need to take precautions, from childhood on, to use appropriate measures (such as a sunscreen with an SPF factor that matches our specific skin type) to shield ourselves from the prolonged exposure to the sun's harmful rays. Sunburn and frequent tanning leave women vulnerable not only to wrinkles but to the far more serious possibility of skin cancer.

Hot flushes, aging skin, and vaginal or bladder discomforts are the most frequent postmenopausal complaints heard by doctors. All of these are generally more flagrant when a woman has lost her uterus and/or ovaries during surgery. In the following sections, we take a look at more insidious conditions that develop in postmenopausal women, with more profound implications.

OSTEOPOROSIS

Osteoporosis is a major health problem facing older women. It is now estimated that *one out of two women will have had one or more osteoporosis-related fractures in their lives*! This adds up to a stunning 1.3 million to 1.5 million bone fractures annually. The cost of this condition—dollars lost in income and those spent on medical care (hospitalization, surgery, physical therapy) and recovery in a nursing home—is an incredible $10 billion annually. The costs in terms of personal damages cannot begin to be quantified when you consider that a woman in her late sixties or early seventies who fractures her hip may end up spending the rest of her life in an institution, dependent on others for her needs and wants. Worse still, one out of every four victims of hip fracture dies within a year because of complications. Despite these sad and frightening statistics, this problem hasn't been seriously tackled. Education regarding prevention is sorely lacking, and therapy once the disease has struck is also inadequate. We have known since 1940 that estrogen replacement therapy is one of the few effective treatments for osteoporosis. Yet for a variety of reasons doctors and patients alike have neglected to aggressively pursue this. Today, only 10 percent of all postmenopausal women are on ERT for this condition.

Worse still is the contribution made by unnecessary hysterectomies to this public health crisis. In 1988 the results of a study made by Dr. Myroslaw Hreshchyshyn and his colleagues were published in *Obstetrics and Gynecology*. The researchers compared the effects of natural menopause with those of hysterectomy and oophorectomy on spine and hip bones. They confirmed that women who have undergone a hysterectomy have "significantly lower" bone densities than healthy women, even when their ovaries remained. One possible explanation is the observation that the ovaries of about one-third of women posthysterectomy cease to function one or two years after surgery. Decline in estrogen has been identified as a major contributing factor to osteoporosis. Furthermore, women who had their ovaries removed showed the most significant and most rapid decline in bone densities of all groups, especially when their ovaries were removed at a younger age. Specifically, women who have their ovaries removed have twice the rate of bone loss as those who experience a natural menopause!

Why the lack of estrogen has such profound effects on a woman's skeleton is an unsolved mystery, because estrogen receptors have never been definitely identified in bone. It may be estrogen's interaction with the parathyroid hormone, and with calcium and vitamin D, that initiates the loss in bone mass. While doctors remain unsure of the exact underlying mechanisms, osteoporosis is clearly a very serious condition with the potential to cripple women. Therefore, a woman should realize the implications when she agrees to undergo a hysterectomy and/or oophorectomy and should never do so when other options exist.

Bone Is a Living Thing

Because of its appearance, many of us tend to forget that bone is vital, dynamic living tissue. Like any other living tissue, it is constantly growing and changing. Bone consists of two types of cells that balance one another to accomplish this remodeling process: *Osteoblasts* are responsible for new bone development and *osteoclasts* mediate bone destruction. As babies, children, and teenagers, we experience a period of rapid bone growth that tapers off by the time we approach our mid-twenties. By our third decade, we experience a shift in bone development—the balance tips toward a reduction in bone formation. Bone that is less dense is obviously more susceptible to injury from even day-to-day activities. When bone mass is decreased to the point that damage such as fractures may occur, osteoporosis is said to be present (see Figure 9.2). Osteoporosis (literally, "porous bone") is characterized by loss of overall bone mass, the deterioration of the skeletal structure, and the increased incidence of fractures—especially in high-risk areas such as the spine, wrists, hips, and ribs. Bones in these areas have more surface area and thus tend to lose bone mass more rapidly than other bones of the body. The period of most rapid bone loss is right after menopause, due to the rapid decline in estrogen levels. This is true whether you experience a natural menopause or one brought on by a hysterectomy.

Who Gets Osteoporosis?

Until menopause, rates of bone loss are similar in men and women. With estrogen decline, women undergo a rapid reduction in bone mass. Osteoporosis affects both the spongy types of bone found in the spine and wrists and the more compact bone found in the long bones of the hips. Relatively soon after estrogen depletion, osteoporosis afflicts the spongy bone, resulting in wrist fractures and spinal fractures. Interestingly, the latter may frequently cause no symptoms. Vertebrae, the bones making up the spinal column, may simply collapse without pain or injury. Eventually, a woman may notice a loss of height or a deformity in the upper back sometimes known as a dowager's hump. Later, as women reach their seventies, the compact hip bones become damaged to the point of fracture. Osteoporosis is a devastating disease with the potential to cause pain, disability, lack of independence, social isolation, and depression.

Osteoporosis affects both men and women, but because men start out with much denser bone, they are less likely to experience its ravages. Most commonly affected are Caucasian or Asian women who have never had children, women who are of short and slender build, those who have a family history of this condition, and those with certain lifestyle habits. Specifically at high risk are women who have diets poor in calcium and high in alcohol and/or caffeine as well as those who smoke frequently and exercise infrequently. And again, early menopause—and especially surgical menopause—are prime causes of osteoporosis. (See box on page 169.)

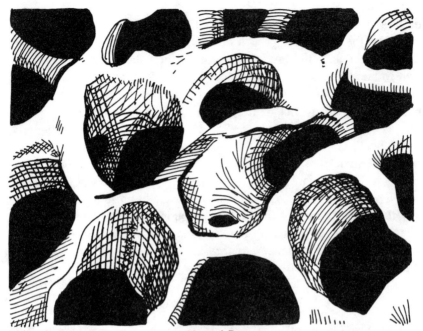

Normal Bone

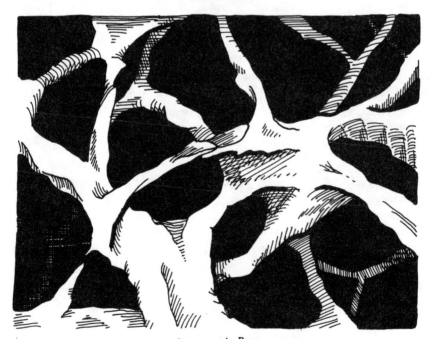

Osteoporotic Bone

Figure 9.2   Normal bone versus osteoporotic bone.

Major Risk Factors for Osteoporosis

You may already be in danger of developing osteoporosis if you

- Are a woman
- Experienced menopause early
- Had a hysterectomy and/or oophorectomy
- Have never had children
- Smoke
- Drink alcohol
- Eat a diet high in caffeine and/or protein
- Eat a diet low in calcium and/or vitamin D
- Exercise rarely or not at all
- Exercise to the extreme of causing your menses to stop
- Are small in stature and slight in frame
- Have thyroid or parathyroid disease
- Have cancer
- Have diabetes mellitus
- Have anorexia nervosa
- Take certain medications, including anticonvulsants or steroids

Making the Diagnosis—Measuring Bone Density

There are no easy, inexpensive, and therefore routine tests to screen for osteoporosis. Regular X rays will reveal the disease only when one-third of the bone has been destroyed. By then, other symptoms have already appeared. However, women at high risk of developing osteoporosis may be selected by their doctors to undergo more accurate diagnostic tests for measuring bone density. The state-of-the-art test for osteoporosis is the *dual energy X-ray absorptiometry (DXA) scan*, which measures bone mineral content in the lower back, hips, and wrists. It is useful to assess women who have risk factors for osteoporosis, those who have already suffered a fracture, and to monitor osteoporosis patients on medication therapy. A DXA scan would be performed before beginning pharmacologic therapy; follow-up scans every two years would provide some insight into whether it is working. CAT scans may also be used to check for osteoporosis, but like DXA scans, they are costly, and in addition, they expose a woman to higher radiation levels.

Finally, blood and urine tests can be performed to track osteoporosis. These tests reflect the cycle of bone buildup and breakdown by measuring the enzymatic (chemical) activity of bone cells that pass into the bloodstream. But these biochemical markers give only an overall picture of what is happening in the entire skeleton and not specifically in the high-risk areas. These tests are costly and are generally performed only by specialists and in clinical trials for new medications. If diagnosis and treatment of osteoporosis are difficult and the effects devastating, then prevention is clearly the key.

Prevention of Osteoporosis

Remembering these caveats can help you begin your battle against osteoporosis early on: First, bone depletion begins to exceed new bone creation when you are only in your thirties and not even beginning to think about menopause. Second, some medical therapies can help restore depleted bone (see the section on New Treatments), but this is a slow and tedious process. Third, while you may have no control over some of your risk factors for osteoporosis, you can make lifestyle changes that will make a difference.

To help lower your risk for osteoporosis, stop smoking, eat a healthy diet high in calcium and vitamin D, and exercise regularly.

SMOKING
Cigarettes have long been called "coffin nails" because of the tremendous number of deaths attributable, at least in part, to smoking. The saying goes that every time you light up, you're adding another nail to your coffin. Scientists know that smokers past menopause are not only at greater risk for osteoporosis, but that their response to estrogen replacement is poorer. This is not only true for bone mineral content. As we shall see in the next section, coronary artery disease is another major health concern for postmenopausal women. Smoking not only contributes to heart disease, but the beneficial effects ERT normally exerts on cholesterol levels are cut in half by smoking.

NUTRITION: CALCIUM AND VITAMIN D
What you eat is as important as what you don't eat when it comes to osteoporosis. At a recent conference sponsored by the European Foundation for Osteoporosis and Bone Disease, experts made the following statement:

> Nutritional intake of elemental calcium is an absolute requirement for bone health, facilitating growth and consolidation and reducing bone loss after skeletal maturity has been reached. The threshold of calcium intake below which bone health is jeopardized varies at different stages of life. . . . It is likely that an ad-

equate calcium intake is necessary for the maintenance of peak bone mass, but it is not known whether a high calcium intake [in] adulthood can contribute to improvements in bone mass. There is a need for studies to address the question of the role of calcium supplementation in the third to fifth decades in women.

It is generally agreed that adequate calcium intake is essential to healthy bones. The problem, however, is that most adult women don't get enough calcium in their diets. This is true for a variety of reasons.

The major source of calcium is dairy foods (see Table 9.2). Unfortunately, some women feel that dairy products are too fattening. Others have an intolerance to milk sugar, or lactose; ingesting milk or cheese causes them to experience uncomfortable gastric problems, such as gas and diarrhea. Others think you don't need to drink milk unless you're a child. The end result is that half of all American women over age fifteen don't consume the recommended daily allowance (RDA) of 800 milligrams of calcium. Indeed, the National Osteoporosis Foundation states that nonpregnant women aged twenty-five to fifty actually need 1,000 milligrams per day; pregnant women and postmenopausal women need another 500 milligrams per day. Worse still, as women age, they absorb less of the calcium that they take in, not only because an older woman's intestinal tract is less efficient, but because vitamin D availability is also less.

Vitamin D is intimately linked to calcium metabolism in the human body. The chief source of this essential chemical is sunlight. Humans synthesize vitamin D within their skin when exposed to the sun; thus, if elderly women remain indoors for most of their days, they may become deficient in this nutrient. The role of vitamin D in the treatment of osteoporosis is very unclear. Some studies have shown its byproducts (not the vitamin itself) to aid in calcium absorption and thus possibly to reduce bone loss and fractures, but the evidence is far from conclusive.

Again, premenopausal women who are not pregnant should try to consume 1,000 milligrams of calcium in their daily diets. The sooner a woman increases her calcium intake, the better, because bone growth is maximal before age thirty. If a woman is past menopause, she needs to increase this to 1,500 milligrams per day. Whether diets high in calcium are really of major benefit to women who already show the ravages of osteoporosis is controversial. Certainly, it can't hurt, and it may help to heal fractures and/or prevent further bone degeneration. As with anything else, be sure not to overdo it, because excessive calcium may cause the formation of kidney stones.

In addition, 400 units of vitamin D are needed every day. This can be accomplished either by being out in the sun for at least fifteen minutes at

Table 9.2   Calcium High Rollers

Food	Calcium (milligrams)	Calories	Fat (grams)
Best Bets			
Yogurt, plain, nonfat, 1 cup	451	126	0.4
Yogurt, plain, low-fat, 1 cup	414	143	3.5
Instant breakfast drink, made with nonfat milk, 12 oz	376	261	0.5
Yogurt, nonfat, sugar-free with fruit, 1 cup	369	122	0.4
Parmesan cheese, shredded, 1 oz	355	129	7.7
Nonfat dry milk powder, 1 oz	349	101	0.2
Yogurt, low-fat, flavored, 1 cup	345	231	2.5
Oatmeal, homemade (½ cup oats with 1 cup 1% low-fat milk)	333	260	5.0
Alba, sugar-free cocoa mix plus calcium, 1 packet	327	62	0.5
Milk, nonfat, 1 cup	316	90	0.6
Milk, 1% low-fat, 1 cup	312	104	2.4
Low-fat frozen yogurt, 1 cup	300	202	4.0
Milk, 2% low-fat, 1 cup	296	121	5.0
Milk, whole (3.3% fat), 1 cup	291	149	9.0
Buttermilk, 8 oz	284	92	2.0
Spinach, boiled and drained, 1 cup	277	53	0.4
Swiss cheese, low-fat, 1 oz	272	51	2.0
Tofu, firm, ½ cup	258	181	11.0
Cheese pizza, 1 slice	220	290	9.0
Premium ice milk, 1 cup	216	242	8.0
Sugar-free cocoa mix, unfortified, small packet	213	48	0.5
Mozzarella cheese, part-skim (low-moisture), 1 oz	207	79	5.0
Sockeye salmon, canned, 3 oz	203	130	6.0
Macaroni and cheese, 1 cup	200	230	10.0
Low-fat processed American cheese, 1 oz	194	51	2.0
Evaporated skim milk, ¼ cup	184	50	0.0
Pink salmon with bones, canned, 3 oz	181	118	5.0
Collard greens, boiled from frozen, ½ cup	179	31	0.3
Waffle, from mix	179	206	8.0*
Ricotta cheese, part-skim, ¼ cup	167	85	5.0
Instant oatmeal, fortified, 1 packet	160	105	4.0
Good Bets			
Vanilla pudding, made with 2% low-fat milk, ½ cup	146	144	2.4
Scalloped potatoes, from recipe, 1 cup	140	210	9.0
Blackstrap molasses, 1 Tbsp	136	43	0.0
Fudgsicle bar	129	91	0.2
Ocean perch, baked or broiled, 3 oz	117	103	1.8
Hot chocolate or cocoa, 1 packet	92	102	1.0
Clams, steamed, boiled, or canned, 3 oz	78	125	1.7
Low-fat cottage cheese, ½ cup	77	82	2.0

Table 9.2 *(Continued)*

Freshwater bass, baked or broiled, 3 oz	73	106	3.4
Rainbow trout, baked or broiled, 3 oz	73	128	5.0
Cream of Wheat or Maypo, ½ cup	62	85	1.2
Shrimp, medium, baked or broiled, 3 oz	55	132	4.4
Pacific halibut, steamed, 3 oz	51	111	2.5
Dungeness crab, steamed, 3 oz	50	86	1.0
Good Bets for Vegetarians			
Spinach, boiled from frozen, ½ cup	139	27	0.2
Turnip greens, boiled, ½ cup	124	25	0.3
Broccoli, cooked from frozen, 1 cup	94	52	0.2
Kale, boiled from frozen, ½ cup	90	20	0.3
Beet greens, boiled, ½ cup	82	20	0.1
Bok choy, boiled, ½ cup	79	10	0.1
Baked beans, homemade, ½ cup	77	190	6.5
Dandelion greens, cooked, ½ cup	74	17	0.3
Small white beans, boiled, ½ cup	65	127	0.6
Navy beans, boiled, ½ cup	64	129	0.5
Great northern beans, boiled, ½ cup	60	104	0.4
Red kidney beans, boiled, ½ cup	58	109	0.1
Fresh spinach leaves, chopped, 1 cup	56	25	0.2

*The fat can be reduced by using a "light" mix or adding less oil than the mix directions call for.

noontime or by drinking vitamin D–fortified milk. Be careful about taking vitamin D supplements because excess amounts can accumulate in body fat and become toxic.

You may be surprised to learn that many foods other than milk and cheese are high in calcium, including beans, tofu, seafood, and green leafy vegetables. You also need to be aware of substances that interfere with the availability of calcium to body tissues. Spinach contains a chemical called oxalate, which binds calcium within the intestine. Diets high in fat and very high in fiber also decrease calcium absorption, as do excess amounts of zinc. Other substances cause calcium to be lost in the urine. One such culprit is caffeine, which is present in coffee, tea, soft drinks, and chocolate. Diets high in salt and protein have a similar effect. Try to cut down on alcohol consumption as well (two drinks per day or less). If all of this sounds like there's nothing safe left to eat, remember that the key to health is trying to have a balanced diet including moderate amounts of protein, carbohydrates, and vegetables with a special emphasis on dairy products.

Don't forget that some medications disrupt calcium and/or vitamin D bioavailability. These include certain drugs taken to prevent seizures and tuberculosis as well as some antacids, blood pressure medications, and steroids used for asthma and arthritis. You should check with your doctor concerning the specific medications you take and whether your dietary requirements may be affected.

If you are unable or unwilling to increase these nutrients in your diet, you can talk to your doctor about supplements. Studies of elderly women have shown a 43 percent decline in hip fractures when they took calcium and vitamin D supplements. It's certainly a good idea to make sure your diet contains adequate amounts of both calcium and vitamin D, but not to consider it to be a definitive treatment for osteoporosis until we have more conclusive knowledge about its effects.

"COUCH POTATO" SYNDROME

Astronauts who have been out in space where there is no gravity for their skeletons to work against have been shown to lose some bone mass. Weight-bearing exercises are believed to stimulate formation of new bone, so it's a good idea to try to incorporate an exercise regimen into your lifestyle. Good gravity-resistive exercises include walking, jogging, dancing, and light weight training. For example, most people can safely walk for thirty minutes at least four times per week. Several words of caution: Be very careful about the type of exercise you attempt if you already have osteoporosis. You don't want to place yourself at risk of falling and sustaining an injury or of undertaking too vigorous a program for your present state of bone health. Consult your doctor first. Likewise, if you have been sedentary and are over age thirty-five, be sure to have a checkup before beginning an exercise program. And whatever your age, begin gradually and build to a moderate pace.

Recent reports by research physiologist Barbara Drinkwater concerning female athletes raise some concerns for going to the other extreme when it comes to exercise. Bone density measurements for some young women who exercise intensely, such as ballet dancers or long-distance runners, resemble those of seventy-year-old women! This is believed to be because they stress themselves to the point of causing hormonal imbalances. Their menses stop and estrogen production declines just as if they were postmenopausal. Thus they begin to develop osteoporosis as if they are postmenopausal as well! Remember, slow and steady wins the race.

Estrogen Replacement Therapy for Osteoporosis

There is definite evidence that estrogen replacement therapy protects women against osteoporosis in several ways. First, ERT will prevent the loss of bone mass and subsequent fractures. For example, women begun on estrogen immediately after having an oophorectomy show almost complete cessation of bone deterioration. The prevention of bone loss seems to hold true even if it is begun ten or fifteen years after the start of menopause.

Second, some doctors believe that even if some damage has already occurred, estrogen can arrest the process and even reverse some of the deterioration. According to Dr. Bruce Ettinger, "Estrogen reverses the bone resorption [thinning] rapidly, allowing the holes that have been formed in the bone to be filled in." It must be stressed, however, that not all doctors agree. Even if the remodeling of bone observed by Ettinger and others is proven out, these reverses are small. Once major changes in a woman's skeleton have taken shape, ERT cannot restore it to its normal form.

That is why prevention is center stage with osteoporosis. Women begun on ERT soon after hysterectomy, oophorectomy, or natural menopause will experience the most dramatic effects. Most researchers believe bone protection will commence at any stage and will continue for as long as a woman continues to take estrogen. Once she stops, however, the effects are unfortunately reversible. This makes ERT a long-term commitment (at least ten years), the pros and cons of which must be evaluated by every woman and her physician individually. In Chapter 8, we talk about how best to come to that decision for yourself.

Most of the studies that have been performed concerning ERT and osteoporosis have examined women taking a particular group of oral estrogen supplements called conjugated equine estrogens. Doses of 0.625 milligrams per day were found to be safe and effective. Larger doses show no added benefit. And it may even be possible to take smaller amounts under certain circumstances. One investigation found that the addition of 1,500 milligrams of calcium per day may cut the necessary dose of estrogen in half. Thus calcium and ERT may go hand-in-hand in protecting women from bone loss.

At present, we don't know enough about the impact other forms of estrogen therapy (i.e., creams and patches) may have on osteoporosis. Nor do we understand exactly how estrogen therapy accomplishes its effects. No one has definitively proven that there are estrogen receptors in bone as there are in the skin, liver, and other organs affected by hormonal changes during menopause. We know only what we observe—that is, if estrogen replacement is begun, calcium absorption, vitamin D production, and calcitonin levels all become normal. (Calcitonin is a hormone that plays a role in bone turnover.) Much more research is needed in this area before the answers to many questions about the role of ERT in osteoporosis may be found.

New Treatments

What if you can't or won't take estrogen and want to protect yourself from osteoporosis? Are there other forms of therapy for preexisting disease? What's new in the area of research and development for this condition? The following is a brief synopsis of alternatives to HRT.

ALENDRONATE SODIUM (FOSOMAX)

Alendronate sodium (Fosomax) is a member of a class of drugs called biphosphonates. This drug was approved for use in 1995 and works by decreasing bone resorption and increasing bone mass of the spine, hip, and total body. Studies published in the *New England Journal of Medicine* reported that women taking this medication have lower rates of hip and spine fractures, less progression of deformities, and less height loss. Clinical trials with this drug demonstrated that women had an increase in the thickness of their spinal bones of 10 percent after about seven to eight months of therapy. The amount of increase in bone density appeared to be dose-dependent. Women on lower doses might not experience a net gain in bone density, but may still be able to maintain the bone stores that they have— neither losing nor gaining bone.

Fosomax is for the use of postmenopausal women who have abnormal DXA tests and/or who have had an osteoporosis-related fracture. It is taken in pill form once a day—a half-hour before breakfast with a full glass of water. Fosomax has been known to cause stomach upset, so it is advised that women taking this medication remain upright and avoid eating or drinking for thirty minutes to minimize this side effect. Aside from gastrointestinal effects, Fosomax seems to pose few problems for women. Women are advised to take calcium and vitamin D supplementation to enhance the effects on bone mass.

CALCITONIN

Like estrogen, calcitonin is a hormone that is believed to act against osteoporosis by retarding bone breakdown. Women taking calcitonin for one year show a 10 to 15 percent increase in bone density. Unfortunately, this effect may be short-lived, with no further improvements observed beyond this period, and regression when treatments are discontinued. In addition, up until recently, calcitonin had several disadvantages that precluded its use for some women. It was available only in an injectable form and as such was extremely expensive, costing roughly $3,000 per year. Injectable calcitonin also caused nausea, vomiting, facial flushing, and a localized skin reaction at the injection site. A nasal spray form of calcitonin called Miacalcin has been available since 1995. Women instill one puff in one nostril every day, alternating between nostrils to avoid irritation to the nasal membranes. Studies have shown intranasal calcitonin to be a safe and effective treatment, in conjunction with calcium and vitamin D therapy.

FLUORIDE

While it does create new bone, fluoride use is controversial for a variety of reasons. First, the bone that is created may be more brittle than normal bone and thus may actually be more prone to fractures! Second, many women are unable to tolerate fluoride's unpleasant side effects, most notably gastric disturbances and inflamed joints. Thus this drug (which is not FDA approved for osteoporosis) has been popular in Europe for many years but never really caught on in the United States. Scientists have recently taken a fresh look at a new formulation of fluoride (Slow Fluoride) that, taken with calcium to add strength to bones, showed promising results in a new study by Dr. Charles Pak and associates published in the *Annals of Internal Medicine* in 1995. In this study of about one hundred women (half on fluoride, half on placebo), Slow Fluoride and calcium taken for four years prevented new spinal fractures and increased bone density both in the spine and hips safely and effectively. Slow Fluoride coats the fluoride in a special capsule that allows passage through the digestive tract without side effects. If approved by the FDA, fluoride will be an inexpensive option for women with osteoporosis. Again, it will be used along with calcium citrate to enhance its effectiveness.

These are some of the treatments that have been shown to have some effect on osteoporosis. For now, however, the best way to overcome osteoporosis is to avoid it entirely by stressing the building of strong bones from a young age through diet, exercise, and the avoidance of unnecessary hysterectomy or oophorectomy. If you are at high risk of succumbing to osteoporosis or have already begun to show telltale signs, you should seriously consider estrogen therapy.

CARDIOVASCULAR DISEASE

Arteriosclerotic disease, which causes a narrowing of the blood vessels supplying necessary oxygen to the heart, brain, and other major organ systems of the body, is responsible for the deaths of one out of every two Americans. It is the leading cause of death in women older than sixty-five. That makes it the most significant health problem facing us today, including all forms of cancer. Interestingly, it has been discovered that women seem to be protected from the ravages of arteriosclerotic disease until they enter menopause, after which their rate of death and disease catches up to men's. As you might imagine, this has significant implications for the woman considering having a hysterectomy and/or oophorectomy.

Arteriosclerosis

The heart is an incredible feat of engineering. A muscular structure containing four chambers, it contracts an average of sixty to eight times per minute every minute of our lives from the time we are still within our mother's uterus to the second we die. With each contraction, blood is forced from the top two chambers into the bottom two chambers and out into the blood vessels that will carry it to all parts of our body. Within this blood are chemicals vital to the maintenance of life, including oxygen, which is the basic fuel for our daily activities. Like any other organ, the heart itself requires oxygen, and the coronary arteries are the blood vessels responsible for servicing the heart's needs.

Arteriosclerosis begins when a type of fat called cholesterol is present in the circulation in excessive amounts. Cholesterol accumulation (among other factors) can cause damage to the vessel walls. These damaged areas attract a particular type of blood cell called platelets, which stick to the area and begin to stimulate the buildup of muscle cells in the lining of the artery. The blood vessel wall eventually becomes narrower and narrower, thus restricting the passage of oxygen-rich blood. When this happens to the vessels supplying the heart, it's called coronary artery disease.

When this process develops gradually, the heart learns to compensate for ordinary activities. Under conditions of physical or emotional stress, however, the heart may require additional energy (and therefore oxygen), which it cannot receive because of the physical limitations of the narrowed arteries. Lack of oxygen causes chest pain known as angina pectoris. This is why, classically, people experience angina when they are upset or exerting themselves in some manner. If a total blockage of a major artery ensues, the portion of heart muscle supplied by that vessel will die. This is what happens during a heart attack.

Likewise, when this process of decreased supply of oxygen to meet the demand occurs in the blood vessels of the brain, transient ischemic attacks (TIAs), or "mini-strokes," take place. Complete blockage or rupture of a blood vessel within the brain is the cause of a stroke. Together, the effects of narrowed blood vessels throughout the heart, brain, and circulation are categorized as cardiovascular disease.

Who Is At Risk?

Women in general seem to have a 10- to 12-year reprieve from the onset of cardiovascular disease, but they catch up rapidly once they enter their middle years. Perhaps the largest and most famous investigation of cardiac disease, the Framingham Heart Study, was undertaken over forty years ago and is still going on today. According to the data collected in Framingham, Massachusetts, "... after 44 years of age, arteriosclerotic disease rises in women at the same rate as in men, and women have the same number of new cardiovascular disease events."

Women, like men, place themselves at greater risk for heart attack and stroke if they (1) smoke, (2) allow themselves to become overweight by eating a high-fat diet, or (3) lead a sedentary lifestyle. The two main medical conditions that also predispose to cardiovascular disease are high blood pressure and diabetes.

Promoting Wellness

As with osteoporosis, prevention of cardiovascular disease is possible. The major emphasis is a reduction in your salt, cholesterol, and fat intake. Salt makes the body retain fluid, and this fluid expands the blood volume. More blood pumping through the same space within an artery (or a narrowed artery when there is arteriosclerosis) causes the blood pressure to rise. This is easy to envision if you think of water running through a hose. When you either turn up the water or narrow the hose, the pressure increases.

The American Heart Association, nutritionists, and others have advocated that Americans reduce the amount of fat and cholesterol in their diets. Remember that the two are not the same. Cholesterol is strictly an animal product. Vegetables are always free of cholesterol and nearly always low in fat. Fruits are also free of cholesterol, but some—such as avocados and coconuts—are extremely high in harmful fats. Fish is generally preferred over red meat in terms of a lower cholesterol content and the presence of certain so-called cardioprotective omega-3 fatty acids. However, shellfish is nearly as damaging as red meat. It is important to familiarize yourself with food labels and types. Armed with this knowledge, you can balance your diet with foods that are low in cholesterol and fats and high in substances that may actually reduce cholesterol levels, such as fiber. Also remember that meat supplies no fiber.

Exercise is also vitally important. It strengthens the heart both directly and indirectly (for instance, by lowering blood pressure). A woman who runs ten to fifteen miles per week, or walks twice that distance, will experience a significant increase in HDL cholesterol levels after about three to four months. Aerobic exercises, in particular, seem to add ten years to a woman's life. Cardiopulmonary fitness tests conducted on sedentary women versus active women showed astonishing results. A woman age forty to forty-nine who worked out regularly was in better shape than inactive women age thirty to thirty-nine. Weight lifting is important in preparing a woman's body for aerobic activities but in and of itself does not show similar effects in terms of improving cardiac fitness. Walking, cycling, and swimming are activities nearly all women can enjoy and profit from.

Furthermore, a recent study published in the *Journal of the American Geriatrics Society* suggested that adding HRT to an exercise regimen would improve lipid profiles (relative levels of overall cholesterol, LDL and HDL cholesterol, and triglycerides; see box below) and cut your risk of death. Hormone replacement coupled with exercise (walking, jogging, and/or stair climbing) complemented each other—resulting in better lipid profiles than either HRT or exercise independently.

Not All Cholesterol Is Created Equal

What is cholesterol?

Cholesterol is a waxy substance that humans both manufacture and ingest. It is a vitally important building block for the body, playing a role in the manufacture of hormones, vitamins, and digestive chemicals, to name only a few.

Where does cholesterol come from?

It is found all over the body, although it is synthesized and stored in the liver. (Dietary sources of cholesterol are found only in animal products, not in plants.) When cholesterol is present to excess, it can clog blood vessels, causing cardiovascular disease.

What's the difference between LDL and HDL cholesterol?

LDL stands for "low density lipoprotein"; HDL signifies "high density lipoprotein." A lipoprotein is a kind of envelope with a protein coat that carries fat and cholesterol through the bloodstream. LDLs contain large amounts of cholesterol that are then deposited in the arterial walls, whereas HDLs contain only small amounts of cholesterol, which they transport away from body tissues to be excreted. Therefore, high levels of LDL cholesterol are associated with an increased risk of coronary artery disease. A high HDL cholesterol level is considered to be "heart healthy."

What's a normal cholesterol level?

Most laboratories consider desirable cholesterol counts to be

TOTAL CHOLESTEROL BELOW 200 mg/dl
LDL CHOLESTEROL BELOW 130 mg/dl

Menopause and Heart Disease

Why should menstruating women have any advantage when it comes to heart disease? Scientists are still unsure, although the obvious clue is that estrogen levels decline dramatically once a woman stops menstruating. When women past menopause are given estrogen supplements, changes occur in their cholesterol levels. Specifically, levels of so-called good cholesterol (protective against coronary disease), known as high-density lipoprotein cholesterol (HDL), rise while harmful low-density lipoprotein cholesterol (LDL) levels fall. Another potential factor may concern the content of a woman's blood pre- and postmenopause. Many women are mildly anemic during their menstruating years. The relatively thinner concentration of their blood (as compared with a man's or a menopausal woman's) may make it less prone to stagnating and thus forming a blood clot. In addition, thinner blood is less resistant to arterial walls and results in lower blood pressure. Lower blood pressure places less stress on the heart and reduces the risk of cardiovascular disease.

Finally, one hypothetical cause of heart disease may be unique to hysterectomy-induced menopause. The uterus produces a substance called prostacyclin, which is critical to blood circulation because it inhibits clotting and dilates, or widens, blood vessels. Once the uterus is no longer present, prostacyclin levels drop. Coronary artery disease may develop more easily in the presence of more viscous blood within a narrower vessel.

Whatever the specific mechanisms involved, postmenopausal women are at definite risk of succumbing to heart attacks and strokes. Furthermore, women who undergo "instant menopause" through the removal of their uterus and ovaries have a risk of arteriosclerosis that develops earlier and to a more serious degree than women undergoing natural menopause. Most, but not all, of the evidence now shows that hormone replacement therapy may restore a woman to her premenopausal state with regard to heart disease risk.

The Heart and Hormone Replacement Therapy

If you are at all familiar with birth control pills, you may be wondering how the estrogen in HRT can protect a woman against cardiovascular disease when the risk of this very same condition is the major harmful consequence of estrogen-containing oral contraceptives. It seems that the answer to this puzzle lies with the fact that HRT relies on totally different types of estrogens (natural versus synthetic) in completely different dosages. According to the American College of Obstetricians and Gynecologists, ". . . estrogen replacement therapy has not been associated with an increased incidence of stroke, embolism, or thrombophlebitis. . . ." Still not convinced? Let's take a look at the evidence concerning post-menopausal women, estrogen, and heart disease.

First, it's important to examine how estrogen replacement might impact on the risk factors for heart disease we have already highlighted, especially cholesterol levels, smoking, obesity, and high blood pressure. Unfortunately, with the exception of its effects on lipids (cholesterol), available data is scarce.

In 1952, the first evidence that women taking oral estrogens had a change in the makeup of their cholesterol was provided. There seemed to be an increase in the HDL component with a decrease in LDL, thus decreasing these women's risk of developing cardiovascular problems. While it has remained controversial whether total cholesterol levels remain the same or decrease, numerous subsequent studies have borne out the original finding that oral estrogen tips the HDL/LDL balance in favor of the heart. In an article published in 1987 by the *American Journal of Obstetrics and Gynecology*, Dr. Bruce Ettinger points out that

> . . . larger doses may reduce the total cholesterol and increase the high density lipoprotein [HDL] by as much as 10%. Although these changes seem relatively minor, reducing a cholesterol level of 250 mg/dl [normal levels are considered to be values under 200 for most labs] by 25 mg/dl should result in a 50% reduction in arteriosclerotic risk.

It is important to note, however, that it is not as clear how other forms of estrogen may influence lipids, particularly those estrogens that are not processed through the liver (which manufactures, stores, and removes cholesterol). Furthermore, when progesterone is added to the estrogen replacement regimen, some of the heart-protective effects may be negated. This seems to depend on what type of progesterone is prescribed by your physician, so be sure to ask about this when considering HRT.

Smoking also alters the effects of estrogens on cholesterol levels. While both smokers and nonsmokers appear to reap the benefits of taking estrogens, smokers can expect to experience only half the response in their lipid levels as nonsmokers.

What about ERT if you are overweight or have high blood pressure? These are again contraindications to estrogen-containing oral contraceptives. Does the same apply here? Apparently, the answer is no. The limited work that has been done appears to show that overweight women who begin ERT actually lose weight, while women who are not overweight do not gain weight. Even more interesting is the fact that women past menopause who do not begin ERT actually gain weight.

There seems to be no association between either high blood pressure or formation of blood clots and ERT. Convincing evidence links birth control pills with all of the above; therefore, your doctor may be reluctant to prescribe ERT if you are overweight or have had a blood clot or hypertension. These factors must be considered on an individual basis while doctors continue to seek conclusive answers through additional research.

Thousands of women on estrogen have been studied in an attempt to determine whether they actually do have fewer heart attacks, strokes, and/or deaths associated with heart disease. Nearly a score of reports has been published, with almost half finding a clear reduction in the risk of cardiac disease for women using estrogens and another quarter finding neither advantage nor disadvantage. These studies looked at women from all walks of life, including nurses, residents of a retirement community, and participants in a health maintenance organization. All in all, most doctors conclude from weighing all the evidence that taking estrogen may even have dramatically beneficial effects, lowering the number of fatal and nonfatal heart attacks by 50 percent! The arguments are even stronger for women who have had their ovaries removed. By some estimates, the death rate is six to seven times higher when estrogen supplements are not taken. (Figure 9.3

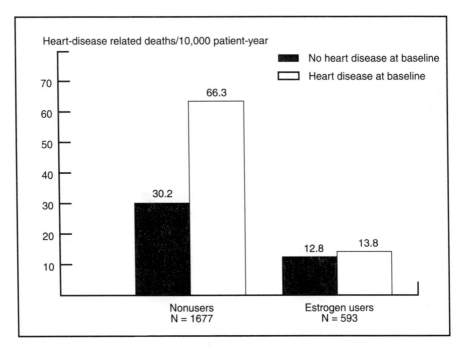

Figure 9.3 Comparison of heart disease–related deaths in users versus nonusers of estrogen replacement.

compares the heart disease–related death rates in users versus nonusers of ERT, according to research from the American Heart Association.)

Thus far we've looked only at the purely physical effects women may anticipate once they undergo menopause. We've seen how these effects can unfortunately be accelerated and exacerbated by premature menopause brought on by removal of the ovaries and (sometimes) the uterus. But what about the less easily identified and quantified psychological effects some women have reported? From my experience, a genuine and serious emotional aftermath exists as well.

THE EMOTIONAL FALLOUT

Hysterectomy, oophorectomy, and their inevitable consequence, menopause, have all been cited as the cause of such psychological symptoms as depression, anxiety, mood swings, decreased memory, impaired concentration, insomnia, fatigue, and decreased sexual desire. Some of these, as we alluded to earlier, may be as a direct result of physiologic (hormonal) changes—most notably hot flushes.

It has been observed that REM (rapid eye movement) sleep, the most restful type of sleep, is decreased and disrupted by the occurrence of nocturnal hot flushes. It comes as no surprise, then, that women who awaken several times a night in a profuse sweat suffer from insomnia, fatigue, and the various consequences of sleep deprivation, such as difficulty concentrating or remembering as well as general moodiness. Estrogen as well as progesterone will help if the underlying problem is purely physical and not the result of a more deep-seated regret or ambivalence toward the loss of one's uterus.

Two common and more extensively studied psychological symptoms linked to hysterectomy and menopause are depression and sexual dysfunction. The chance of developing these conditions is a serious concern raised by women both before and after they undergo hysterectomy. Thus it is important that we carefully examine both with respect to how commonly they actually strike, and in terms of what can be done to minimize any damaging effects they may cause.

Depression

The first reports of depression following pelvic surgery were published in the *American Journal of Psychiatry* in 1941 by Dr. Lindemann. Later, a term was even coined for it: posthysterectomy syndrome. Various studies pointed not only to a higher rate of admissions to psychiatric hospitals but also a generally higher rate of emotional problems (two to three times higher) among women who had undergone a hysterectomy as compared with women having their gallbladders removed. Mental illness, it seemed, was a common side effect of hysterectomy, afflicting by some estimates as many as 70 percent of women postoperatively! Yet this knowledge did not deter physicians from subsequently performing millions of these operations each year.

More recently, these conclusions have been challenged in some circles, and the subject has become more controversial. However, many hysterectomy patients that I have seen tell me a story of severe loss—of grief over the loss of an organ. Because of this, I routinely counsel patients contemplating this surgery and ask them how they would feel if they had a hysterectomy. Instead of having patients tell me that they really don't know how they might feel, I get one of two answers. Some patients say that they will experience significant grief and that they don't want to lose their uterus even if it is causing them pain, even if it is malfunctioning, even if having less invasive surgery now (i.e., myomectomy) might mean they will need more surgery later. These patients will certain experience a significant loss if faced with a hysterectomy. However, some women with whom I discuss the possibility of uterine conservation reply that they don't feel that it's necessary to save their uterus. After all, they argue, what do they need it for? They're not going to have children. They're experiencing a troublesome problem, such as a large fibroid, that may continue to cause problems at a later date, and they want to have the uterus removed. These women are probably not going to become depressed, because they want to have the surgery. Thus it's my judgment that the cause of this depression is a mind-set.

From my experience, eight out of ten women want their uterus preserved! Therefore, it's vitally important for any woman contemplating hysterectomy to consider that she may become depressed and to be aware of what factors increase her risk.

How Will I Feel?

Joan is a forty-two-year-old mother of two grown sons. When Joan's second son was born, she was treated briefly for a bout of postpartum depression. Married to a truck driver who is often on the road for long periods of time, Joan finds herself with frequent slots of empty time on her hands now that her job of full-time wife and mother is not as demanding. Despite the necessity of sacrifices and strict budgets, Joan says she and her husband both felt it was more important for her to be home for the children and to manage the household than to have a career of her own. Except for recent times, Joan always felt that she was "too busy" to get involved with outside activities, such as charitable works or the PTA.

Two months ago, Joan underwent a hysterectomy with removal of both of her ovaries for a fibroid tumor. Her gynecologist had told her that he was alarmed by its unusually large size and advised that surgery be scheduled immediately. Joan and her husband heard the words "large tumor" and agreed that she would have the surgery scheduled two weeks later. She still feels incapable of resuming some of the work around the house, and because of the nature of his job, her husband is not really available to help her. Furthermore, Joan is concerned that he is distancing himself from her—for example, by deliberately volunteering for overtime and for particularly extensive road trips.

Lately, especially when no one is home, Joan finds herself lying in bed until noon and hanging around the house in her nightgown. She feels listless and seems to "cry at the drop of a hat." She feels very unattractive and finds that she is sometimes grateful that her husband has found other things besides her to occupy himself with.

Some women do become clinically depressed after a hysterectomy; therefore, all should think twice about the need for their hysterectomy. They should weigh any available alternatives and take into consideration how they will feel when it's all over. If you have made a well-thought-out, well-informed decision, have allowed yourself and your family adequate time and resources to prepare for hysterectomy, and feel that having the operation is the best choice in your situation, you will significantly minimize any depression.

Joan's story highlights some of the risk factors and symptoms associated with posthysterectomy syndrome. First, she had a history of a previous bout with depression after the birth of her second son. She has opted for a very traditional role—one in which childrearing was central to her concept of herself. Now her children are grown, and she must readjust and consider how she will spend the rest of her life. Right now, she is bored and has too much time on her hands. Furthermore, Joan's partner is both physically and emotionally distant from her. He seems to view her along traditional lines as well, and both Joan and her husband may have certain notions about hysterectomy and sexuality that are influencing their attitudes and behavior. Finally, Joan had the operation within a month of her initial doctor's visit, which left them little time to be properly educated or emotionally prepared. All of these factors have resulted in Joan clearly demonstrating some of the symptoms of depression, including feelings of listlessness, sadness, decreased sexual desire, and a disinterest in day-to-day life. (See box on page 187.)

* * *

Symptoms of Depression

Depression is a common side effect of hysterectomy. The American Psychiatric Association lists these major symptoms of depression. If you answer yes to at least five of the questions and have had these feelings for at least two weeks, you should seek help. Fortunately, talking with a therapist and/or taking medications can be extremely helpful in treating and curing depression.

1. Are you in a depressed or irritable mood most of the day, nearly every day, as indicated by your own feelings or as observed by others?

2. Do you have a markedly diminished interest or pleasure in all, or almost all, activities most of the day, nearly every day, as indicated by your own feelings or the observation by others that you are apathetic? Have you noticed that you don't feel much better, even temporarily, when something good happens?

3. Have you experienced a significant weight loss or weight gain (e.g, more than 5 percent of your body weight in a month), or a decrease or increase in your appetite nearly every day?

4. Do you suffer from insomnia or excessive sleepiness nearly every day? Are you waking up two hours (or more) earlier in the morning than usual?

5. Have others noticed that you are excessively agitated or lethargic nearly every day?

6. Do you feel fatigued—without any energy—nearly every day?

7. Do you have feelings of worthlessness or excessive or inappropriate guilt nearly every day?

8. Do you feel unable to concentrate or make decisions, nearly every day, in your own judgment or by the observation of others?

9. Do you have recurrent thoughts of death (not just fear of dying), recurrent suicidal ideas (without a specific plan)? Have you made a suicide attempt or a specific plan for committing suicide?

David Youngs and Thomas Wise, two experts in the field of psychological aftereffects following elective hysterectomy, tell us that the main issues for women facing hysterectomy include the loss of reproductive function, the loss of menstrual function, and threats to sexual function. Women who have hysterectomy before they have completed their families are bound to be severely depressed. Even women for whom menstruation may have been fraught with problems may express depression once they no longer experience what most women view as a natural, valuable, and uniquely female function. But of all the risk factors that have been cited to cause postoperative depression, one of the most common revolves around a woman's fear of sexual changes. In research that studied women's anxiety related to hysterectomy, the women who became depressed afterward were those who believed that hysterectomy would make them fat, prematurely old, less interested in sex, and less desirable to their husbands. Thus how a husband deals with his wife's surgery is just as important to her mental health and self-esteem as are her own feelings. In an article published in 1984 in the journal *Psychosomatics*, Drs. Martine Lalinec-Michaud and Frank Engelsmann wrote:

> A woman who is insecure about her attractiveness is more prone to expect that her husband might lose interest in her following the removal of her womb. Indeed, the husband's reaction has a strong influence on the woman during this sensitive period of time . . . strong support from the spouse may greatly facilitate a healthy rehabilitation period.

Unfortunately, men have been known to reject their wives, and marriages have broken up more often, as a result of this surgery than from, for example, gallbladder operations. Clearly, both men and women have to understand what's happening and come to grips with their feelings to avoid these consequences.

What You Can Do if You Need a Hysterectomy

Experts believe that you can avoid or minimize posthysterectomy depression if you heed the following guidelines.

BE SURE TO TELL THE GYNECOLOGIST WHAT YOU WANT

Make sure you trust your gynecologist, and get a second opinion wherever possible so that you are comfortable that having a hysterectomy is the course you wish to pursue in the treatment of your gynecologic problem. If you truly don't want to lose your uterus under any circumstances, seek that second opinion with a physician who is sensitive and attuned to alternative methods that help women to avoid hysterectomy whenever at all feasible. Research has shown that women suffering from non-life-threatening problems (which might have been solved another way?) were much more likely to become depressed than those who expressed a profound sense of relief that a dreaded condition (e.g., cancer) was now behind them. Certainly, hysterectomy will solve the medical problems and the anatomical defects in a woman with fibroids, for instance, but the body is more than a uterus! It is a human being with a human mind and emotions. Therefore, the gynecologist has to be concerned with finding out from a woman exactly what this surgery would mean to her, and to understand that even if a woman is prepared to take certain (non-life-threatening) risks to preserve her self-image, he or she must respect and comply with her feelings. As long as a woman understands that the alternative to hysterectomy she has selected may not offer a permanent solution or a 100 percent cure, then she is entitled to make the choice.

To sum up, here are the words of Drs. Youngs and Wise:

> Social, psychological, and even cultural aspects of gynecologic surgery inevitably involve three principal individuals—the patient, her family, and the physician. Each plays a critical role in the successful outcome of any surgical treatment. A healthy comfortable relationship among all participants provides the best insurance against misunderstanding, regret, and subsequent untoward psychological sequelae.

Researchers Hackett and Weisman further reinforce my admonition concerning the absolute necessity of finding an understanding physician: "... [U]nless it is understood that the interpersonal dimension operates within both patient and doctor, the patient is apt to be considered identical with the diseased organ and the surgeon a totally disengaged technician."

GET "THE FACTS, MA'AM, JUST THE FACTS"

It's important that you and your partner sit down with your doctor or nurse and receive a clear explanation of the operation, the recovery period, and any long-term side effects. Review any concerns you may have and dispel any erroneous fears based on what you may have heard from others. Be sure that you ventilate all of your feelings and get concrete and realistic answers to all your questions. Various studies have shown that even women who did receive information before their operations may not have benefited very much. In follow-up interviews, they complained that the advice was too broad. For example, they may have been told not to lift anything heavy, but not exactly what the weight limitations were or for how long they should maintain the restriction. Or they were sung the praises of hysterectomy ("you'll be a new woman in six weeks"), when their recovery actually took much longer in many cases. In addition, discussions were sometimes described as too short, with too much information presented for them to assimilate in one sitting. Try to have several conversations with your doctor or nurse, and make sure you keep in contact until all of your

questions have been answered. Finally, even health professionals may be reluctant to bring up the topic of sex, so don't you be. Remember, uncertainty
in this area was one of the most frequently cited risk factors for depression.

Allow Yourself Time to Do the Work of Worrying

Unless it's an emergency, take time to prepare yourself for the surgery—
emotionally and physically. You may not think that having a hysterectomy
will represent a big change in your life, but it very well may; and people
generally need time to psych themselves up. Studies show that women who
knew at least a month ahead that they were going to lose their uterus had
much lower rates of depression than women who had very little advance
warning. Consider the advice of Dr. Lalinec-Michaud and Dr. Engelsmann:

> Women having a hysterectomy after short notice experienced a
> significantly greater pre- and postoperative depressive morbid-
> ity. It is conceivable that women need some mourning time to
> adjust to the thought of an important intervention such as hys-
> terectomy, which is perceived as a loss and a threat to the in-
> tegrity of self-concept. Allowing sufficient time prior to the
> operation, when possible, would help facilitate better pre- and
> postoperative adjustments.

Have Frank and Open Discussions with Your Partner

Discuss openly what this surgery represents to both of you. Don't minimize or deny your feelings. If you fear that you may somehow become less
attractive or less sensuous, gaining reassurance from your partner that he
doesn't feel this way can make all the difference. If your partner worries
that you may be "altered"; that because you can no longer get pregnant,
you're no longer as appealing somehow; or that you'll lose interest in sex,
it's imperative that you work this out. You may both need to seek professional help either to set the facts straight or to cope with these feelings.
(See box on page 191.)

Realize That You Are Not Alone and That Help is Available

Look for help from support groups (see the Appendix), psychotherapy, and
medication should you become depressed. Remember that feeling depressed
from time to time is quite normal. It turns into actual pathology only when
these feelings are so severe and prolonged that they interfere with your ability to deal with daily life. If you find that you are feeling sad, worthless,
anxious, unattractive, ill, helpless, or hopeless (especially to the point of
contemplating suicide), and if these feelings pervade every facet of your
life from work to leisure for two weeks or more, it's time to seek help.

Guide to Choosing a Therapist

Many women and their families may desire and benefit from some form of counseling or psychotherapy when faced with the issue of hysterectomy. The following are some commonsense tips to help you find the therapist or counselor who best suits your needs.

1. **Check credentials.** Myriad titles and levels of training must be sifted through when trying to find an appropriate match for your particular wants and needs. Common titles include the following:
   - *Psychotherapist.* This title may imply any level of training drawn from a variety of backgrounds. No laws govern who may use it; it is a self-imposed label. A psychotherapist may be a psychiatric nurse specialist, a social worker, even someone with a college degree in psychology. While it's most important that the individual you consult has experience in your problem and that you feel comfortable with him or her, this is a case of caveat emptor (let the buyer beware). Be sure that your psychotherapist has the proper training and qualifications.
   - *Psychologist.* Anyone using the title of psychologist must have a doctoral degree (Ph.D.). These individuals undergo approximately five years of postgraduate work, and their specialty is "talk therapy." There are two types of psychologists—both have equal levels of training, but with a different focus. A "clinical psychologist" has the title Psy.D. and training that emphasizes clinical experience. The traditional Ph.D.'s training is split between clinical and academic aspects.
   - *Psychiatrist.* A psychiatrist is a physician (M.D.) specializing in emotional illness. He or she has completed medical school and done a residency in psychiatry. Unlike other types of therapists, a psychiatrist is the only one licensed to prescribe and dispense medications (but in some states, psychiatric nurse practitioners are permitted to do this). Therefore, if you require antidepressants, or perhaps hormones (some psychiatrists would prefer to leave that to your gynecologist), a psychiatrist may be a good choice. Remember, too, that a reputable psychologist who determines that your problem requires medication will refer you to a psychiatrist with whom he or she collaborates. You can then continue to see your nonphysician provider for talk therapy and the doctor for medication.

Guide to Choosing a Therapist (*Continued*)

2. **Consider cost.** Psychotherapy can be a costly undertaking and is not always covered by medical insurance plans. If this is the case for you, it's worth looking into community mental health centers or teaching clinics affiliated with major universities that have doctoral programs in clinical psychology. The latter utilize students who are supervised by advisers in the therapy they provide. Both resources usually offer low-cost counseling or have a sliding fee scale based on your ability to pay.

3. **Get referrals from reliable friends and colleagues.** They may be able to offer good leads and a starting point—one preferable to the Yellow Pages. Just remember that a therapist may consider that there is a conflict of interest if he or she is also seeing your friend. However, even if you can't be taken on as a client by this therapist, he or she can refer you to someone else. It's a good networking move.

4. **Shop around.** Call to make an appointment with one or more therapists that you are considering. Honestly explain that you wish to have a trial session with them to see if they can help you with your problem. In the trial session, go with your gut feeling about this person. Consider the following:

   - Do you feel at ease with this person? Of course, there is always a certain amount of unease. After all, this is your first interaction with a stranger with whom you will be sharing the intimate feelings and details of your life. A good therapist will recognize this and should be able to put you at ease.

   - Is the therapist talking too much? In the first one or two sessions, you should be doing most of the talking. Early on, it is the role of the therapist to be the interviewer. He or she should be eliciting information about you and the details of your problem by asking questions. It is too soon for the therapist to be analyzing the situation, drawing conclusions, and advising you on major life changes. Beware if the therapist is talking more than he or she is listening.

   - Do you feel as though this person really "hears" you? In other words, does the therapist seem to understand and empathize? You should feel that a strong alliance is possible with this individual—that he or she will be helpful and trustworthy.

   - Do you perceive that the two of you have the same or similar value systems? This is especially important when choosing a sex therapist. You have to feel that the therapist is not being judgmental, so that you can be totally open and honest.

Guide to Choosing a Therapist (*Continued*)

- What is the therapist's clinical orientation or vision of psychotherapy? In other words, does the therapist's mode of treatment involve a long-term commitment (e.g., an analytic approach) or does he or she subscribe to a more short-term model of therapy? Does the type of practice fit in with the type of problem you need help with? For example, someone who wants to quit smoking would be better off with a behavioral therapist than engaging in years of psychoanalysis.

5. **Consider a female therapist.** For some women, because of the nature of the problem, having another woman to talk to is essential; for others it is not. Go with what feels right to *you*.

6. **Ask the therapist if he or she has any experience with problems related to menopause or hysterectomy.**

7. **Once in therapy, evaluate the following:**
   - Are you making progress? Remember that change doesn't happen overnight, but you should get a sense that things are moving forward. If they are not, honestly consider whether it's because of you or because of the therapist. Don't hesitate to bring it up in your sessions—this may certainly change the pace of things.
   - Is the therapist acting inappropriately? If you feel that a therapist's behavior is somehow improper (especially a sex therapist's behavior), discontinue seeing that therapist and consider whether you need to report him or her to the proper authorities.

8. **Remember that therapy and therapists are not "forever."** If you feel you have made a mistake in choosing someone, you can always make a change.

Keep Active and Lead a Healthy Lifestyle

This is generally good advice for any situation. Specifically here, if a woman has other diversions and interests not tied to mothering, she may not feel all is lost when her uterus is lost. In addition, from a practical point of view, exercising regularly will help you to avoid the weight gain you may fear to be a consequence of hysterectomy. Exercise also increases the levels of beta endorphins, chemicals in the brain that are known to reduce pain and increase feelings of general well-being. Plenty of rest and good nutrition are also essential to dealing with stress. High-protein foods, such as milk, also improve sleep and the sense of well-being. Avoiding the urge to take solace in empty calories can help prevent weight gain, which can make depression worse.

SEXUALITY—
HOW MUCH PSYCHOLOGY?
HOW MUCH PHYSIOLOGY?

Roughly 40 percent of women report a decrease in sexual response after hysterectomy. Contributing to these troublesome statistics are a variety of physical and emotional factors. As pointed out in the previous section, issues concerning sexuality are often the prime suspects in posthysterectomy depression. Women (or their partners) who believe they will experience sexual problems actually have more sexual problems as the result of a self-fulfilling prophecy. It's vitally important that women and their sexual partners confront their fears and raise their concerns in this area in order to minimize this effect. Ellen and her husband had tremendous difficulties in this area after her hysterectomy:

When I was thirty-eight, I had a hysterectomy for severe bleeding. I was being so tortured by my periods that I didn't even think about any down side to the surgery. Something else, however, was going on in my husband's mind. Naturally, I didn't think much about Ed's lack of sexual advances immediately after my operation. After all, he was just being cautious and considerate. The doctor had told us to avoid intimacy during the recovery period until I returned for my postoperative examination.

It was after I was given the green light that I noticed something was wrong. The first time, it really hurt. I told myself that I must have been nervous. Still, I could see that there was a change in Ed's manner and behavior. He must also be nervous, I mused.

I decided to discuss the matter with my gynecologist, since I was concerned that something might have gone wrong with the surgery. He told me that absolutely nothing had gone wrong and that having your uterus removed had nothing at all to do with sex. Sex, he said, was in your mind, not in your uterus. He told me not to listen to what other women said about how their sex lives changed after hysterectomy. These were old wives' tales and I was a modern woman. He said that I was probably sending subliminal messages to my husband that were affecting his performance as well.

In other words, it was all in my head, it was all my fault; it was from a mythology built up by women, and the sooner I realized all of this, the sooner I'd get well. In fact, I discovered that it was my husband's fears and beliefs that were at the root of the problem. He came from a very old-fashioned family and his value system prevented him from enjoying sex with a neutered woman. Unfortunately, he did not consciously confront his feelings beforehand, and it took us some time to work through this in therapy afterward.

Ellen's gynecologist's words are very reminiscent of those of W. Gifford-Jones, M.D., author of the 1977 book, *What Every Woman Should Know about Hysterectomy*:

> Gynecologists would have stopped doing this operation years ago except where it was life-saving if a significant number of their patients ended up in the psychiatrist's hands. The same thing applies to cases one hears about where women have a change of heart sexually toward their partners. Lamentably, many problems exist in the bedrooms of the nation long before a hysterectomy is required. To some women, the operation therefore presents an excellent out. Yet it is impossible to change a healthy woman's posture towards sex, and women who have always enjoyed sex will have the same liking for it after the operation.

It's easy to blame a woman for what may be a natural decline in sexual interest and activity with the approach of middle age, especially if she's undergone menopause or hysterectomy. The renowned Dr. Kinsey discovered in his research on human sexual response that both men and women experience parallel decreases in sexual interest beginning around the fourth or fifth decades of life, and these were unrelated to a woman's hormones. A century before, Dr. Colombat L'Isere had pronounced sex dead after menopause:

> It is the dictate of prudence to avoid all such circumstances as might tend to awaken any erotic thoughts in the mind and reanimate a sentiment that ought rather to become extinct . . . in fine, everything calculated to cause regret for charms that are lost, and enjoyments that are ended forever.

Today, by contrast, many postmenopausal women who see themselves as free of the concerns of pregnancy and contraception may say that they enjoy sex more than ever. This includes a substantial number of American women who have had a hysterectomy. However, in cultures where sexuality is valued only as long as reproduction is possible, the loss of libido and the perception of painful intercourse unfortunately is very common. In Nigeria, for instance, 70 percent of women report being totally abstinent even before they pass their first decade beyond menopause. Their male partners generally take new wives with whom they can have more children; not long after this, the first wives experience a loss of desire and other negative feelings concerning sex that cannot be coincidental.

Again, it's vital to consider and confront how you and your partner might feel about your sexuality after a hysterectomy. Instead of dismissing or ignoring any negative feelings, come to terms with them before having a hysterectomy, or better yet, don't have it done!

Does all of this mean that if a woman experiences sexual dysfunction after a hysterectomy, it's all in her mind? Not by a long shot. As already discussed, decreased estrogen causes physical changes in the genitalia, including a shortened, less elastic, and drier vagina. The surgery may also alter the vagina because of the formation of scar tissue, or because it has been shortened or tightened. Furthermore, many women say that during an orgasm, their uterus contracts, causing pleasurable sensations. If a uterus is no longer present, it obviously cannot contribute to orgasm. The absence of the cervix may also change a woman's sensation during intercourse and contribute to painful sex because it can no longer produce lubrication when she becomes aroused. Finally, removal of the ovaries removes one important source of testosterone—the hormone believed to play the greatest role in sex drive. The surgery results in immediate discomfort, of course, but of greater concern are permanent changes in a woman's pelvic anatomy that may be a lifelong consequence resulting in lifelong sexual problems.

Unfortunately, these physical changes may not have easy solutions. A gynecologist may brush them off and say that artificial hormones or lubricating jellies will compensate. While these aids can be helpful, they are no substitute. As author Susanne Morgan, who herself has had a hysterectomy, points out, lubricating jellies restore wetness to the vagina, but they do nothing to replace the lack of arousal that would have stimulated the vagina to become lubricated in the first place. As far as hormone replacement therapy is concerned, she also makes an important point:

> Articles implying that estrogen replacement makes everything exactly as before are misleading. No one tries to convince a diabetic that the insulin shots are exactly the same as the insulin produced naturally in the body. A diabetic knows that he or she must take care not to get out of balance and that the insulin simply moderates some of the changes. Even if menopause were an "estrogen deficiency disease" as some people try to portray it, taking estrogen could not totally prevent all changes or adjustments.

So again, don't have a hysterectomy unless you are convinced that there is no other solution to your problem. And don't expect (even if you are told to the contrary) that you will feel exactly the same as before. You may feel the same; you may feel better; or you may feel worse.

Preserving Your Sexual Feelings

Sex therapists Masters and Johnson (among others) believe that sexually active women avoid the atrophic changes normally caused by a decline in estrogen. No one is sure why this use-it-or-lose-it phenomenon occurs, although a couple of theories were put forth earlier in this chapter.

In addition, hormone replacement is helpful: Estrogen restores vaginal tone and lubrication. Progesterone may decrease depression (thus enhancing sexual interest). And testosterone increases libido, although it must be given judiciously because of its negative side effects.

A water-based lubricant, such as K-Y Jelly, can provide artificial moisture in the vagina that will decrease painful penetration. While this doesn't substitute for natural arousal, by preventing pain it may stimulate your body's own natural processes, promoting relaxation and enjoyment.

Finally, to help you cope with purely psychological barriers to sexual enjoyment following a hysterectomy or menopause, a number of books and other resources are available on the subject. (See the Appendix for a listing of resources.) Most of all, remember that staying sexy is a state of mind that needs to be nourished by spontaneous emotion and experimentation.

* * *

The onset of menopause for some women may be associated with noticeable changes in the functioning of their bodies. This is especially true for those whose menopause is sudden and dramatic due to the removal of their uterus and ovaries.

The universal changes that occur, of course, include the end of menstruation and the ability to bear children. For some women, this marks the beginning of a new era of sexual freedom and the pursuit of a new lifestyle that might mean, for example, embarking on a career unencumbered by family responsibilities. Other women, especially those whose personal satisfaction and self-esteem are intimately linked with their ability to bear children, may experience some depression with the loss of these functions.

Women undergoing menopause may also notice a range of other effects, including hot flushes or changes in their skin and sexual organs, to name a few. No two women experience menopause in the same way. It's important to recognize that you may have none or all of these symptoms, and that many of the symptoms are transient as your body adjusts.

10

ALTERNATIVE AND ADJUNCT THERAPIES AND THE ROLE OF NUTRITION

The best doctors in the world are Doctor Diet, Doctor Quiet, and Doctor Merryman.

—Jonathan Swift

Thus far, we've discussed the main conditions that have led women—sometimes unnecessarily—to have or be advised to have a hysterectomy. We've seen that conventional medicine now can offer you a modern array of surgical and nonsurgical options to manage the problems that no longer mandate such a radical approach. But it is also vitally important to acknowledge the alternative therapies that could offer you a totally different approach and/or an adjunct approach to what you may be doing now. Alternative therapies and adjunct therapies speak to the tremendous role that you play in steering the course of both the management of your condition and your recovery.

WHAT IS ALTERNATIVE MEDICINE?

I wish I could give you a simple definition for what is meant by alternative medicine, but the simple fact is that no single definition or explanation exists for what has grown to be a huge industry with a huge following in the United States today. In 1993 the *New England Journal of Medicine* reported that 34 percent of 1,539 participants in a large-scale study had used alternative therapies in the past year—often paying out of pocket ($10.3 billion!) because such therapies were not covered under traditional health insurance plans. If this study conducted by Dr. Eisenberg and associates from Beth Israel Hospital in Boston took traditional doctors by surprise (most respondents had not informed their regular doctor of their alternative treatment), recent times have seen the field blossom with

199

books, internet websites, and medical practices that offer this kind of assistance (see Appendix). Indeed, Burton Goldberg's *Alternative Medicine—The Definitive Guide* lists forty-three different types of alternative therapies.

The following is meant to be a brief and simple introduction to the various major types of alternative therapies that might be beneficial to you if you have fibroids, endometriosis, abnormal bleeding, or prolapse, or if you are experiencing some of the posthysterectomy or postmenopausal symptoms discussed earlier in the book. It is not possible or appropriate within the scope of this book to offer an exhaustive list of all of the possible alternative therapies. Keep in mind, too, that what we often consider alternative medicine in the West is mainstream medicine elsewhere—for example, acupuncture. You might want to consider exploring how your problems might be treated if you were from another country or had a different cultural background.

Several main underlying themes seem to be threaded through the web of alternative medicine regardless of where or how it is practiced:

- Practitioners of alternative medicine do not consider their treatments to be quackery. They are based on scientific principles regarding how the body functions, but differ from conventional therapies in that they are frequently "natural" versus pharmacological.
- Unlike allopathic medicine (the traditional training of the majority of doctors in the United States and other Western industrialized countries), alternative therapies focus on prevention rather than cure. Allopathic doctors see a symptom or illness and work toward reversing that illness; alternative practitioners emphasize a healthy lifestyle to head off illness and then attempt to use the body's own processes and powers to heal itself if illness does occur.
- The whole person—mind and body and the interplay between the two—is considered in alternative therapy practices. Specialization or focusing on one organ or body system is deemphasized. Instead, the emphasis is holistic.
- Adjunct therapies are frequently aimed at reducing stress, boosting your immune system, improving your nutritional status, inducing a state of relaxation, alleviating pain, improving your outlook, and maintaining hope; thus, they may work well on chronic conditions.
- The influence of the environment—both the individual's lifestyle and the global environment—are important in the explanation of the causes of illness and disease as well as in their prevention and cure.

Deciding on an Alternative Therapy—Things to Consider

If you do decide to pursue alternative therapy, it might be wise to see it as an *adjunct* rather than a true *alternative* to conventional therapy—depending on the severity of the problem. In addition, as with selecting a traditional physician, it is important to research the health care provider and his or her type of treatment carefully before undergoing it. Here are some things to consider if you are thinking about trying alternative or adjunct therapies:

- None of the adjunct therapies should hurt you (except for the minor pain sometimes involved with massage). They should not contain so-called secret ingredients, be extremely expensive, or promote the exchange or exposure to blood or body fluids that are not your own (due to the risk of contracting hepatitis, AIDS, or other infectious diseases).

- Don't be fooled by credentials. Names followed by impressive-sounding initials do not indicate that the treatments offered are safe or effective. Be aware that credentials other than M.D. (such as N.D., naturopathic doctor) are licensed and monitored differently from state to state. Try to investigate the doctor to make sure that he or she is currently legally permitted to practice and that no complaints have been filed against him or her by former patients or the authorities.

- Let your conventional doctor know about the alternative therapies you are seeking so that the therapies can complement rather than conflict with one another. Don't be embarrassed to bring the subject up. You have a right to pursue an alternative or adjunct therapy. If your doctor is resistant to or critical of your decision to pursue an adjunct therapy, try having a frank and open discussion with him or her. Most clinicians will accept (if perhaps not sanction) your use of alternative medicine as long as they see that it is safe and won't conflict with their plan of care. On the other hand, if an alternative or adjunct therapy involves a procedure that is invasive, painful, or requires that you take some kind of "medicine," it is important that you discuss this with your regular doctor to assure that there is no reason, in his or her opinion, that this would be unwise for you.

- Carefully and thoroughly investigate the therapy you wish to try. Ask questions and read everything you can on the subject. Always ask to see studies published in respected journals that back up the use of the therapy in question. Never rely solely on testimonials.

- Beware of promises that seem too good to be true. Beware of big promotions for products or treatments.

- Remember that therapies offered in other countries may not be covered by consumer protection laws in the United States.
- Costly therapies should be suspect. If you are asked for thousands—even hundreds—of dollars, be suspicious. Remember that your health insurance may not cover what is considered alternative or experimental treatment.
- Don't fall prey to extreme forms of therapy or ones that make outrageous claims. For example, be wary of "mega" anything. Excessive amounts of a product or treatment of any kind is probably worthless at best, and potentially harmful at worst.
- Be cautious of those who would try to talk you out of seeking a second opinion about a particular therapy.
- Discuss the adjunct therapy with your loved ones. Get their opinions and enlist their help, if necessary.
- Consider your options, cost, the time necessary, and so forth before choosing a therapy.
- Dedicate yourself to learning and practicing the therapy if this is appropriate.
- Monitor your progress.
- Remember that you can stop and change to another therapy at any time.

In this chapter, we will focus on nutrition, natural hormones, and herbs as well as traditional Chinese medicine, such as acupuncture, because these seem to be the alternative therapies most appropriate to female health.

NUTRITION AND DISORDERS OF THE REPRODUCTIVE SYSTEM

It is currently believed that girls begin to menstruate when the estrogen levels in their bodies reach a critical level and that estrogen production depends on body fat content. This may be the reason that female athletes who train intensively or women suffering from eating disorders such as anorexia nervosa stop getting their periods when their body weight (and their body fat content) drops below that critical level. High-fat diets, which are very common in Western industrialized countries such as our own, allow the body to manufacture greater amounts of estrogen. Add to this the fact that commercially-produced meat and poultry are often supplemented with hormones and it is not surprising to discover that diet can play a role in helping or hindering some of the conditions we are concerned with in this book.

The Role of Diet in Fibroids and Endometriosis

According to Ronald Hoffman, M.D., a traditionally trained physician and noted expert in the field of alternative medicine who is the medical director of the Hoffman Center for Holistic Medicine in New York City, fibroids have an unpredictable response to diet depending on how many fibroids are present and how large they have grown. Fibroids will sometimes respond to "a very clean and natural diet," but sometimes they continue to grow despite adherence to dietary restrictions. Hoffman believes that the genesis of fibroids, as well as that of many other disorders that often threaten women with hysterectomy (such as endometriosis and dysfunctional bleeding), stems from a common origin—that is, some form of hormonal dysregulation. In other words, under the influence of unbalanced hormonal stimulation, several common problems—from breast disease to excess menstrual bleeding—might develop. According to Hoffman, overgrowth of the uterine lining (endometrium) is associated with too much estrogen and not enough progesterone, with fibroids and endometriosis both being conditions that can develop as a reaction to this so-called hyperestrogenic state. Excess estrogen, as we've said before, is related to fat intake and body weight, so let's take a moment to consider obesity.

OBESITY

Sadly, the latest information about obesity in this country is that for the first time in our history, more Americans are overweight than are of normal weight. Overweight women tend to have heavier menstrual periods and more gynecological problems. Says Dr. Hoffman, "Caloric overnutrition results in the production of excess fat cells, and excess fat cells or enlarged fat cells tend to amplify the effects of estrogen." Furthermore, when you eat livestock that has been fed hormones and antibiotics to make it more appealing to our tastes and thus more marketable (fatty meat is tastier than lean meat), those antibiotics may have an effect on how the intestinal flora native to your digestive tract can process both the foreign hormones you take in as well as the estrogen you produce yourself. This results in a net increase in the amount of estrogens your body contains.

Losing weight and trying to decrease your intake of xenoestrogens (estrogens that are foreign to the body, such as those in water contaminated with chlorinated hydrocarbons, DDT, PCB residue, or those in commercially produced meats and poultry) are two ways to avert or stem the common problems of fibroids, endometriosis, and heavy menstrual flow.

However, there is also a genetic link to both fibroids and endometriosis. Fibroids, for example, can arise in any woman—thin or obese—as a result of a genetic mutation that need only affect a single cell! Hence, it is also important to understand how to manage fibroids and endometriosis from a nutritional vantage point—even if you are thin and even if you already have these conditions and cannot hope to prevent them by trying to alter your environmental influences. Here is where prostaglandins may come into play.

PROSTAGLANDINS AND EICOSANOIDS

Prostaglandins are naturally occurring chemicals within the fatty acid chemical family that have an effect on the actions of certain hormones within the body as well as on the uterus, other muscle tissue, and blood pressure. They are probably most noted for their role in the body's inflammatory response. Eicosanoids are the chemical building blocks for prostaglandins within our bodies. Like cholesterol, there are good and bad prostaglandins and good and bad eicosanoids; also, some are manufactured within the body and some are taken in via diet. According to Hoffman, "A new notion is that we can determine the direction of our prostaglandin chemistry by our diets. The way that this happens is through managing obesity and thereby controlling excess insulin [a key digestive hormone]. Insulin has a gatekeeper effect on the way that good eicosanoids or bad eicosanoids get manufactured in the body." Hoffman points out that another way to mediate eicosanoids in the body is through the types of oils and fats that we consume in our diet. A diet that is heavily weighted toward animal fat will cause the proliferation of bad eicosanoids; these are pro-inflammatory eicosanoids and may increase susceptibility to inflammatory conditions such as endometriosis—and may even create a greater tendency toward cancer. According to Hoffman, eating foods that contain the essential fatty acids that are the building blocks of good prostaglandins may reduce the severity of symptoms of endometriosis and fibroids, for example. Foods that provide good eicosanoids include vegetable and fish oils; examples of foods that contain bad eicosanoids are beef fat and margarine.

To reiterate, the idea is to favor the production of good prostaglandins or eicosanoid building blocks for prostaglandins, which are the chemical messengers for inflammation. The aim is to turn off the pro-inflammatory messengers that can contribute to the signs and symptoms of endometriosis and fibroids.

HORMONE-RICH FOODS AND HORMONE-MODULATING FOODS

Certain foods actually have hormonal effects because they contain hormones. We touched upon this earlier in our discussion of meats and poultry that contain hormone residues. In addition, dairy products are prone to contain hor-

Dr. Hoffman's Nutritional Strategy to Help Manage Fibroids and Endometriosis— A Pesco Vegetarian Diet

Dr. Ronald Hoffman, alternative medicine and nutrition expert, suggests that you might be able to help decrease the effects of endometriosis or fibroids by following these nutritional guidelines.

- Eat a diet that is low in fat and calories.
- Decrease the amount of meat and poultry you eat, emphasizing instead soy and other beans as substitute protein sources and as sources of beneficial eicosanoids.
- Use only vegetable oils in cooking. Studies show that women from Mediterranean countries who consume large amounts of olive oil appear to have less heart disease and lower incidences of breast cancer. The latter seems to suggest that this may be due to the estrogen-modulating effect of these oils.
- Choose fish as a source of protein and of omega-3 oils, which possess beneficial chemicals to decrease negative prostaglandin effects.
- Increase your lignans, found mostly in beans, fresh fruits, and vegetables (see Table 10.1).
- Select a diet that is high in fiber and whole grains, but low in refined flour products such as some breads and pastas. Fiber assists the digestive tract to process estrogens and eliminate excess amounts from the body. Excess estrogen levels can make you prone to fibroids, endometriosis, and breast and uterine cancers.
- Reduce dairy consumption because milk products contain hormonal residues. Substitute other sources for calcium; for example, green leafy vegetables, fortified soy products, and sardines.
- Increase magnesium intake. According to Dr. Hoffman, 90 percent of his patients with endometriosis are magnesium deficient, which contributes to the painful menstrual cramping associated with this condition. Magnesium can be taken orally, or in more severe cases, by injection or even intravenously.
- Increase iron consumption in the form of fish, beans, and leafy green vegetables, and/or supplements in the dosages recommended by your doctor if you have heavy menstrual bleeding and anemia as a result of your fibroids or endometriosis.
- Cut down sugar to less than 10 percent of your total caloric intake because sugar may interfere with estrogen metabolism in the liver.

Table 10.1 Common Fruits and Vegetables That Are Rich in Phytoestrogens and Boron

	Phytoestrogens		
	Isoflavonoids	Lignans	Boron
Fruits			
Apples	✓		✓
Apricots			✓
Avocados			✓
Bananas			✓
Berries	✓		
Blueberries			✓
Gooseberries			✓
Red raspberries			✓
Strawberries	✓		✓
Cantaloupe			✓
Cherries, sour			✓
Citrus fruits	✓		
Grapefruit			✓
Oranges			✓
Figs			✓
Grapes	✓		✓
Mandarin oranges			✓
Mangoes			✓
Papaya			✓
Peaches			✓
Pears		✓	✓
Plums		✓	✓
Vegetables			
Asparagus		✓	✓
Beets		✓	✓
Bell peppers	✓	✓	✓
Broccoli	✓	✓	✓
Brussels sprouts			✓
Cabbage	✓		✓
Carrots	✓	✓	✓
Cauliflower		✓	✓
Celery root			✓
Chinese cabbage			✓
Corn			✓
Cucumbers	✓		✓
Dandelion leaves			✓
Eggplant	✓		
Endive			✓
Garlic	✓	✓	
Leeks		✓	

Table 10.1 (*Continued*)

	Phytoestrogens		
	Isoflavonoids	Lignans	Boron
Lettuce, all types	✓		✓
Iceberg		✓	
Onions		✓	✓
Radishes			✓
Rutabagas			✓
Snow peas		✓	
Spinach			✓
Squash	✓	✓	
Sweet potatoes		✓	✓
Tomatoes	✓		✓
Turnips		✓	✓
Yams	✓		

mones because they are mammary secretions of animals. Some foods contain chemicals that can actually modulate the hormonal effects of other foods. These chemicals comprise two basic groups: isoflavones and lignans.

Isoflavones are found mostly in beans and particularly in soybeans. Two key isoflavones that block the harmful effects of hormones present in foods are genislein and diadzin. These may actually lower excessive levels of estrogen and slow the development of fibroids and severe endometriosis. It is particularly interesting to note how isoflavones function in the body, because in spite of the fact that they block estrogen at the level of the uterus and the breast (to decrease or delay diseases in these organs), these same chemicals may actually act as pro-estrogens on bones! Hoffman believes that isoflavones may enhance bone strength and help fight osteoporosis because they are capable of "duality of action."

The second major group of hormone modulators are called lignans. They are present in a high concentration in flax seed and are also found in other seeds and vegetables. Lignans can alter the intestinal circulation of estrogen and thus can actually moderate the amount of estrogen that gets circulated back into the bloodstream and reabsorbed into the intestines. In other words, they act to sweep out excess estrogen in the body.

Finally, studies reveal that women who eat vegetarian diets produce less estrogen than do women who consume both meat and vegetables. This may be due to the added effects of increased fiber and decreased fat. In addition, it appears that increasing exercise reduces the risk of many diseases, including those related to the reproductive tract. Thus, we come back to the generally holistic nutritional advice to increase one's intake of fruits, vegetables and fiber; increase water consumption (preferably from an environmentally safe source); and increase exercise to attempt to minimize the inflammatory effects of such conditions as fibroids and endometriosis as well as the painful symptoms that accompany them.

ALTERNATIVE THERAPIES
FOR DISORDERS
OF THE REPRODUCTIVE SYSTEM

Traditional Chinese Medicine

Much more ancient than allopathic Western medicine, traditional Chinese medicine has been used by billions of people over thousands of years. It is a completely different approach to healing and may complement your current therapeutic regimen. The underlying philosophy of Chinese medicine is to look at the person as a whole, including his or her diet and lifestyle, and try to ascertain what imbalances might be present that may have led to illness. Unlike Western medicine, which identifies a *symptom* and treats that symptom with one or more standard protocols, Chinese medicine uses a variety of treatments specific to the patient and based not on the symptom itself but on what the Chinese physician identifies as the underlying *cause* of that symptom. For example, according to Dr. Oreste Pelechaty, who is director of the Aloha Holistic Health Clinic in Millburn, New Jersey, and board certified in acupuncture and Chinese herbology, endometriosis may be treated very differently in different women because the cause may be different. The restoration of harmony and balance of the opposing forces of yin and yang (respectively, the female passive and male active principles in nature), and the reestablishment of the body's life force—its *Qi* (commonly written as "chi" and pronounced "chee")—are of paramount importance.

The examination of a patient by a traditional Chinese practitioner involves careful observation—of the skin, tongue, pulses, body language, voice, and general demeanor. It also involves careful listening to ascertain clues to what in that person's diet, job, activities—even the weather—has caused the disharmony. Treatment may include one or more of the following: herbs, special diets, acupuncture, massage, and/or special exercises to clear blockages in one's energy channels, or *meridians*, and to get the *qi* flowing smoothly once more.

ACUPUNCTURE
Used mostly to aid in various kinds of pain relief, acupuncture involves the use of presterilized, disposable needles of varying lengths that are passed through the skin at specific points along the body (meridians) that corre-

spond to specific organs of the body. The free end of the needle is then twirled, or it can be used to conduct small electrical currents to the preselected point, thereby inducing a type of anesthesia that in turn relieves or reduces pain. It is thought that acupuncture may accomplish this by triggering the release of endorphins, which are substances produced by the brain and believed to be the body's natural painkillers. A person undergoing acupuncture is awake at all times. It is said to be painless, but each individual responds differently. Treatments can take place once or twice a week for months, or can be limited to a single visit. The length of time per treatment also varies. Some states require a practitioner to be licensed; others require certification by the National Commission for the Certification of Acupuncturists. Costs vary greatly. If performed by an M.D., acupuncture may be covered by some medical insurance policies.

According to Dr. Hoffman, acupuncture can be helpful in the treatment of fibroids because this therapy acts on the nervous system, which controls circulation; and it is pelvic congestion (the stagnation of blood within the pelvic organs and their associated blood vessels) that is responsible for the discomforts of fibroids, including the pain and sensation of heaviness some women experience. Likewise, acupuncture may work to alleviate the painful cramping associated with endometriosis.

However, it is important to have an evaluation by an experienced practitioner of Chinese medicine who will tailor a multifaceted care plan directed at what he or she sees as the underlying disharmony and which may include acupuncture as only one aspect of the treatment plan.

Herbal Medicine

Herbal medicine is the most ancient form of healing as well as the one with the closest ties in many ways to "modern," or conventional, allopathic medicine in that the pharmaceutical products prescribed by traditional doctors have almost always been derived from plants. Herbal medicine, also known as botanical medicine, involves the use of plant products, most commonly in the form of teas, tablets, tinctures, oils, and ointments to treat a particular symptom. Herbs are generally weaker but gentler in their actions than traditional pharmaceuticals, resulting in a more gradual improvement but with fewer side effects. But don't be lulled into complacence when using herbal formulations—they can be very potent and even poisonous. Proper and effective use requires consultation with an herbal specialist and demands the same respect afforded the use of traditional medicines. Some of the more common herbs used to treat uterine disorders include *dong quai*, motherwort, vitex, and life root.

Homeopathy

Based on the theory that "like cures like," homeopathy bolsters the body's natural protective mechanisms using "medicines" made of very dilute solutions of herbs, minerals, and animal and plant extracts. A specific substance is diluted to achieve the smallest amount of the substance that can be used to control a symptom. Only one substance or medicine is used at a time. Homeopaths believe that physical symptoms are the body's way of trying to cure itself—for example, a runny nose and sneezing is the body's way of curing its own cold; thus, if you cause the nose to run, you help the body to cure itself. No school is accredited to teach homeopathy exclusively. Education is generally via national study groups. Some homeopaths are medical doctors with added training. As with traditional Chinese medicine and herbal medicine, it is best to see a homeopathic doctor to receive a prescription for the most effective treatment for your specific situation.

Though not traditional homeopathy, in that it does not employ traditional homeopathic remedies drawn from the original pharmacopeia, Dr. Hoffman and others are attempting to treat endometriosis by utilizing principles related to this field. Specifically, based on the theory that endometriosis may be an allergic reaction to the body's own tissues—in other words, a case of the body's immune system turning against itself in an *autoimmune* response—minute doses or weakened versions of estrogen and sometimes progesterone are administered to help the body to build up a tolerance to its estrogen. This is similar to people receiving trace doses of what they are allergic to—in the form of allergy shots—to desensitize them to a full-scale exposure. Some alternative medicine experts believe that the origin of this autoimmune, or allergic, response that in turn triggers the inflammatory condition of endometriosis is actually a systemwide yeast infection—one much more extensive than the one that causes common vaginitis. According to Dr. Hoffman, "The yeast triggers an aberrant response by the immune system called 'molecular mimicry'—it is as if the immune system is trying to lash out and fight the yeast but this process may cause a cross reaction with certain tissues. Studies have shown higher levels of anti-ovarian antibodies (chemicals produced by the body's own defense system but designed to take action against its own ovaries) in women who have chronic yeast infections. So yeast may be the basis of certain immune disregulatory reactions that may contribute to female problems which seem to be a marker in patients who have endometriosis."

NUTRITIONAL STRATEGIES FOR MENOPAUSE

We have already devoted a good deal of discussion to nutrition and menopause, including the need to increase calcium and vitamin D and to reduce fat and cholesterol in order to ameliorate the harmful duo of osteoporosis and heart disease that seems to accompany estrogen decline (see Chapter 9). Also, several books on the subject of nutrition and menopause have been published. (See Suggestions for Further Reading at the end of this chapter.) This section will therefore serve as a general overview of the subject, with a special focus on nutrition as an alternative therapy for menopause, particularly when a woman is unable or unwilling to go the traditional route of HRT.

It is interesting to note that whether we are talking about fibroids, endometriosis, heart disease, osteoporosis, hyperlipidemia (elevated cholesterol), diabetes, or menopause, the nutritional advice is almost always the same! You can't seem to go wrong if you eat a well-balanced diet that emphasizes fiber, fish, fruits, and vegetables over sugar, caffeine, salt, refined flour products, meats, and poultry (especially dark meat).

The Effect of Menopause on Metabolism and Digestion

As the body ages, its ability to absorb certain essential vitamins and minerals from the digestive tract decreases, thus necessitating the need to increase one's intake of these nutrients to compensate. At the same time, metabolism slows, making it easier and easier to gain weight, but harder and harder to lose it. According to nutrition expert Elaine Moquette-Magee, menopausal women face the dual challenge of having to get more of many nutrients with fewer calories! In her book, *Eat Well for a Healthy Menopause*, she outlines what she calls "the 10 Diet Commandments for a healthy menopause":

1. Eat at least one phytoestrogen-rich food every day. (See Table 10.1.)
2. Eat at least one boron-rich food every day because boron is helpful for bone metabolism. (See Table 10.1.)
3. Limit your intake of caffeine, soft drinks, and alcohol—and drink plenty of water.
4. Eat about 150 percent of the RDA for the vitamins and minerals you need more of as you age.
5. Eat many small meals throughout the day, and eat lightly at night.

6. Eat at least two calcium-rich foods every day, preferably ones also high in vitamin D.
7. Eat several antioxidant-rich foods every day. (See Table 10.1.)
8. Eat no more than 20 to 25 percent of your calories from fat.
9. Eat 20 to 30 grams of fiber every day, from a variety of different foods.
10. Limit your intake of sodium and sugar.

PHYTOESTROGENS

You may already be familiar with this term, but in case you're not, a phytoestrogen is simply a plant—sometimes an herb—that has estrogenlike properties. Whether or not you're on HRT, increasing your phytoestrogens will be beneficial. Because the most common type of estrogen supplement prescribed by medical doctors, Premarin, is a byproduct of a horse, not a human, it may cause some adverse effects in some women. If you find this to be the case for you, you may opt to try phytoestrogens instead. If you still experience menopausal symptoms after trying phytoestrogens, you may need to seek out pharmacies (see Appendix) that will specially compound natural estrogen and progesterone for you, or ask your doctor to switch you to non-animal estrogen formulations.

Hundreds of different plants, including apples, strawberries, grapes, peppers, broccoli, sweet potatoes, and carrots, have estrogenlike properties (see Table 10.1). However, soybeans have the most pro-estrogenic effects, that is, they are thought to be potent enhancers of the estrogens already present in the body. As discussed in a previous section, soy products (such as tofu and tempeh) can modulate hormonal influences, helping to minimize harmful effects (such as the increased incidence of inflammatory conditions like endometriosis) while at the same time maximizing the beneficial effects (such as decreasing the signs and symptoms of menopause).

BORON

Adding boron to the nutritional picture supplements the beneficial effects of phytoestrogens. Boron is a trace mineral that appears to bolster estrogen levels in postmenopausal women by as much as double! It also decreases calcium excretion. Plums, peaches, and strawberries are among the foods highest in boron, but you can refer to Table 10.1 for a complete list of boron sources.

CAFFEINE, SOFT DRINKS AND ALCOHOL

We've already talked about how caffeine and phosphates in soft drinks leach calcium from bones, thus predisposing a woman to osteoporosis. But caffeine can also cause insomnia and anxiety and contribute to the common mood disturbances postmenopausal women notice most. Likewise, alcohol can depress the nervous system and, like sodas, add unwanted calories. In addition, some forms of alcoholic beverages (particularly red wine and beer) can trigger headaches, which again are a common problem for postmenopausal women.

ANTIOXIDANTS

Oxidation in the body can lead to changes that we associate with cancer and aging. Vitamin C, vitamin E, and beta-carotene are antioxidants believed to be capable of blocking the cell-damaging effects of oxidation. Many fruits and vegetables are great sources of these vitamins (see Table 10.2). Of course, in addition to adding antioxidants to the system, it is equally important to avoid things that promote damaging oxidation, such as cigarettes, alcohol, and exposure to excessive sunlight.

Table 10.2 Antioxidant-Rich Foods

Food Serving	Antioxidants Provided*		
	Beta-Carotene	Vitamin C	Vitamin E
Fruits			
Cantaloupe, cubed, 1 cup	✓	✓✓	
Grapefruit, half		✓	
Grapefruit sections, canned, ½ cup		✓	
Guava, half		✓✓	
Kiwi		✓✓	
Mango	✓✓	✓✓	
Mango slices, ½ cup	✓	✓	
Orange		✓✓	
Orange sections, fresh, ½ cup		✓	
Papaya, half		✓✓	
Papaya slices, ½ cup		✓	
Strawberries, whole or sliced, ½ cup		✓	
Tangelo		✓	
Tangerine sections, ½ cup		✓	
Vegetables			
Beet greens, boiled, 1 cup	✓	✓✓	
Bell pepper, red, half		✓✓	
Bell pepper, yellow, half		✓✓	
Bell pepper, red, chopped, ½ cup		✓✓	
Broccoflower, steamed, 1 cup		✓✓	
Broccoli pieces, cooked, 1 cup		✓✓	
Broccoli pieces, raw, 1 cup		✓✓	
Brussels sprouts, boiled, 1 cup		✓✓	

(Continued)

Food Serving	Antioxidants Provided*		
	Beta-Carotene	Vitamin C	Vitamin E
Butternut squash, baked and mashed, ½ cup	✓✓		
Butternut squash, baked cubes, 1 cup	✓✓	✓	
Carrot	✓✓		
Carrot, raw, grated, ¼ cup	✓		
Carrot slices, steamed, ½ cup	✓✓		
Cauliflower, boiled, 1 cup		✓✓	
Cauliflower, raw, 1 cup		✓✓	
Chicory greens, raw, chopped, 1 cup	✓		
Chili peppers, raw or canned, ¼ cup	✓	✓✓	
Chinese cabbage, steamed, 1 cup		✓✓	
Dandelion greens, boiled, 1 cup	✓✓		
Dandelion greens, raw, 1 cup	✓		
Dock/sorrel greens, raw, chopped, 1 cup	✓	✓✓	
Green pea pods, cooked, 1 cup		✓✓	✓
Hubbard squash, baked cubes, 1 cup	✓✓		
Hubbard squash, boiled and mashed, ½ cup	✓		
Kale, boiled, 1 cup	✓✓	✓✓	✓
Kohlrabi, boiled, 1 cup		✓✓	
Lamb's-quarters, boiled, ½ cup	✓✓		
Mustard greens, boiled, 1 cup	✓	✓	
Peas, raw, 1 cup		✓✓	
Peas and carrots, boiled, 1 cup	✓✓		
Pumpkin, boiled from fresh, ½ cup	✓✓		
Pumpkin/squash mix, canned, ½ cup	✓✓		
Snow peas, steamed, 1 cup		✓✓	
Spinach, boiled, 1 cup	✓✓		
Spinach, fresh, chopped, 2 cups	✓	✓	
Sweet potato, baked without skin	✓✓		✓
Sweet potatoes, canned, ½ cup	✓✓		✓
Swiss chard, boiled, 1 cup	✓	✓	
Turnip greens, boiled, 1 cup	✓✓	✓	
Winter squash, baked cubes, 1 cup, or mashed, ½ cup	✓		
Yams, orange, mashed, ½ cup	✓✓		
Fruit and Vegetable Juices			
Apple juice (plus vitamin C), 8 oz		✓✓	
Cranberry juice cocktail, low-cal or regular, 8 oz		✓✓	
Grapefruit juice, 8 oz		✓✓	
Orange juice, 8 oz		✓✓	
Pineapple juice, 10 oz		✓	
Pineapple juice (plus vitamin C), 8 oz		✓✓	
Strawberry juice, 8 oz		✓✓	

Food Serving	Antioxidants Provided*		
	Beta-Carotene	Vitamin C	Vitamin E
V-8, low-sodium or regular, 8 oz		✓✓	
Yellow passion fruit juice, 8 oz	✓		
Beans and Bean Products			
Lima beans, cooked from dry, 1 cup			✓
Soybeans, cooked from dry, 1 cup			✓✓
Tofu, ½ cup			✓
Nuts and Nut Butters			
Almonds, 1 oz			✓✓
Almond butter, 2 Tbsp			✓
Filberts/hazelnuts, 1 oz			✓
Soybeans, roasted, ½ cup			✓
Sunflower seed butter, 2 Tbsp			✓✓
Sunflower seed kernels, roasted, 2 Tbsp			✓✓
Oils			
Almond oil, 1 Tbsp			✓
Cottonseed oil, 1 Tbsp			✓
Hazelnut oil, 1 Tbsp			✓
Rice bran oil, 1 Tbsp			✓
Safflower oil, 1 Tbsp			✓
Sunflower oil, 1 Tbsp			✓✓
Other			
Mayonnaise, 1 Tbsp			✓

*Food servings that provide at least 50 percent of the RDA for a given antioxidant are followed by a check mark in that column. Food servings that provide around 100 percent of the RDA for a given antioxidant are followed by two check marks in that column.

ALTERNATIVE THERAPIES TO DECREASE THE SYMPTOMS OF MENOPAUSE

HOT FLASHES AND FLUSHES

Women who eat a diet that is high in soybeans seem to suffer less from hot flashes and other symptoms of menopause. This may be because soy products are among the highest in phytoestrogens. Increasing phytoestrogens, boron, magnesium, and vitamin E (take at least 300 IU per day) while decreasing alcohol and caffeine should be beneficial for alleviating hot flashes. In addition, try herbs such as *dong quai,* ginseng, motherwort, vitex, black cohosh, life root, and garden sage to temper hot flashes.

VAGINAL DISCOMFORT

Topical estrogen and vitamin E creams applied directly to the vaginal tissues will help to keep them supple, as will continuing to engage in regular sexual activity (if you are able). And, as mentioned in Chapter 9, discomforts caused by the thinning and drying out of the vaginal tissues can also be aided by using such water-based lubricants as Astroglide, K-Y Jelly, or Surgilube.

BLADDER SYMPTOMS

A variety of nonsurgical and nonhormonal techniques were introduced in Chapter 7 to help with the problems often brought on by a decline in estrogen, such as uterine prolapse and urinary incontinence. Urinary tract infections are also common in menopausal women, because changes in the tissues that line the bladder can make you more susceptible to bacterial colonization. To prevent bladder infections, drink plenty of fluids, particularly water and cranberry juice, and remember to urinate frequently, especially before and after intercourse. Finally, it is believed that the herb yarrow is helpful for bladder problems related to menopause.

NERVOUS SYSTEM SYMPTOMS

Menopause can usher in many different effects on the nervous system; the less desirable ones include headaches, insomnia, fatigue, problems with concentration and memory, and a variety of mood disturbances—from anxiety to depression. Alternative medicine clinicians experienced in helping menopausal women cope with these symptoms can prescribe phytoestrogens and a variety of helpful herbs, including ginseng, vitex, black cohosh, life root, and garden sage.

RECOVERING FROM A HYSTERECTOMY— NATURAL HORMONE THERAPY

It's been emphasized here time and again that estrogen and progesterone are necessary to many of the functions of the female body, and that a decline—particularly a decline in estrogen—can have detrimental effects on many organ systems, especially the skeletal and cardiovascular systems. Some women do not want to take HRT, or they cannot take it because of a history of either breast or endometrial cancer, gallbladder disease, liver disease, high blood pressure, blood clots, migraines, or a host of other conditions that make it unwise to be on traditional regimens. While phytoestrogens in the form of dietary supplements and/or herbs are much less potent than conventional supplements, they are somewhat beneficial, although more in terms of modulating the side effects of menopause than its more serious consequences such as osteoporosis.

Disogenin is a plant product found in wild yams, soybeans, and various herbs that can be converted to progesterone and, like other forms of natural progesterone, may have fewer unpleasant side effects than the synthetic progestins currently prescribed by most physicians.

If you don't have any medical contraindications to HRT, but are bothered by the side effects that it can produce, you might want to try to take natural estrogen and progesterone. Some are commercially available; others are available only in formulas obtained through specialized pharmacies, such as the Women's International Pharmacy (see Appendix). Three brands of natural human estrogen are currently available commercially and can be prescribed by your gynecologist: Estrace comes in tablets and vaginal cream; Estraderm and Climara are skin patches that slowly release the estrogen into the body over a given period of time.

Again, posthysterectomy women should assure that they take in adequate amounts of calcium, magnesium, boron, and vitamins D and E. A diet that is low in fat and sugars and supplemented by such essential fatty acids as gamma linolenic acid, which can be found in evening primrose oil, will help to keep you at the peak of health.

* * *

Bear in mind that the alternative medicine practitioners I consulted, as well as the literature written on the subject, emphasized that severe disorders (large fibroids, advanced endometriosis, etc.) could not be reversed (except in very rare instances) by alternative medicine practices. However, trying these various methods may certainly be appropriate for you as an adjunct to your present treatment plan, as an alternative if you are not a candidate for more conventional management of your condition, and/or if you simply want to approach your problem from a variety of vantage points. Alternative therapies emphasize healthy ways of eating, exercising, and inducing relaxation—of generally slowing down, thinking about the poisonous substances (like nicotine and alcohol) you may be ingesting—and treating your body with more respect than is usual in our fast-paced and stressful lifestyle.

Suggestions for Further Reading

Alternative Medicine—The Definitive Guide by the Burton Goldberg Group (Future Medicine Publishing, Inc., 1994).

Eat Well for a Healthy Menopause by Elaine Moquette-Magee (John Wiley & Sons, Inc., 1996).

Tired All the Time: How to Regain Your Lost Energy by Ronald L. Hoffman, M.D. (Pocket Books, 1995).

HOPE FOR THE FUTURE

Women truthfully are unique mammals, carrying, feeding, and nurturing their young; surviving a greater percentage of the time in utero and earlier in the neonatal period and, ultimately, living longer than men.

—DEREK LLEWELLYN-JONES, 1971

I'd like to end this book on a hopeful note. Much of what has been explored here pointed to a history that was not always encouraging. What was said was not always positive; sometimes it was downright critical. However, this book is being published on the threshold of a new millennium that holds a bright and promising future for women suffering from a variety of conditions that at one time would have mandated hysterectomy.

In 1900 Dr. George Engelmann spoke before a meeting of the American Gynecological Society. This forward-thinking man's words could not have rung any truer then than they do today:

> We seem to have attained the apex of surgical achievement but there are peaks beyond, new fields to conquer. . . . We cannot safely rest on past achievements; we must struggle onward. . . . Along the lines of extirpation, we can no longer advance; we must look to preservation, to the conserving of the function, and this I believe to be the surgery of the twentieth century.

Much work still needs to be done in order to fulfill the aspirations so eloquently stated by Engelmann. In writing this book, I hope to educate women about their bodies. Specifically, it is my goal to contribute to raising women's consciousness concerning hysterectomy—a procedure that I believe to be performed far too frequently without knowledge or consideration of the alternatives.

In addition, I hope that physicians will also become more enlightened, emphasizing research and development in the areas of medical and surgical alternatives to hysterectomy. This book not only describes utilization of lasers, electrocautery, and refined surgical instruments via the laparoscope and the hysteroscope to offer a safer and less invasive option than traditional surgery, but also points to improvements in medical therapy for all gynecological concerns from teenage endometriosis to menopausal symptoms.

219

Finally, I hope that we will soon see the day when the crisis in health care brought about by a shortage of financial resources will force the medical community and those responsible for administering our health insurance system to recognize that the less invasive alternatives to hysterectomy are much more cost-effective. For example, while "illness-oriented" health care plans presently cover the cost of a hysterectomy, they do not generally pay for health maintenance procedures such as Pap smears. Yet this simple, inexpensive test has prevented countless numbers of hysterectomies through early cancer detection. Likewise, insurance companies do not reimburse for many procedures that are considered "too new and experimental," even though studies performed by myself and others have proven their safety and efficacy. Moreover, these procedures may frequently be performed as ambulatory surgeries, saving the costs of hospital beds and nursing care, not to mention time lost from work as a result of a shortened recovery period.

I was trained in a big city hospital where a premium was placed on the number of hysterectomies you did and not on how good you were at preserving someone's uterus. We often did not anticipate, nor did we consider, the tremendous impact such surgery would have on a woman's life—on the way in which she and her loved ones might view her once her reproductive capabilities had been taken away from her. The way you are trained stays with you for a while, and old habits die hard. In the seventeenth century, Joseph Addison said, "When men are easy in their circumstances, they are naturally enemies to innovations." However, the time has come for all of us—patients, doctors, health care administrators—to look toward the future. Today, 50 percent of all hysterectomies can be eliminated by critical evaluation, another 40 percent by advanced medical and surgical techniques. We must recognize that alternatives to hysterectomy benefit each and every one of us. The time to change is now.

HELPFUL ORGANIZATIONS

Alternative Medicine

American Association of Acupuncture and Oriental Medicine
4101 Lake Boone Trail, Suite 201
Raleigh, North Carolina 27607
919-787-5181

This is a nationwide professional organization of acupuncturists who meet acceptable standards of competency and will refer you to a member professional in your area.

American Association of Naturopathic Physicians
2366 Eastlake Avenue, Suite 322
Seattle, Washington 98102
206-323-7610

Maintains a nationwide network of naturopathic physicians and will be able to refer you to an accredited or licensed practitioner in your area.

American Botanical Council
P.O. Box 201660
Austin, Texas 78720
512-331-8868

This is a nonprofit research- and education-oriented organization offering publications on various herbal medicines.

International Foundation for Homeopathy
2366 Eastlake Avenue, Suite 301
Seattle, Washington 98102
206-324-8230

Provides a referral list of homeopaths, and offers courses for lay people and professionals.

National Center for Homeopathy
801 North Fairfax, Suite 306
Alexandria, Virginia 22314
703-548-7790

Provides a referral list of homeopaths, and offers courses for lay people and professionals.

Cancer/Smoking Cessation

The National Cancer Institute Office of Cancer Communications
National Cancer Institute
National Institutes of Health Building 31, Room 10A24
Bethesda, Maryland 20892
Toll-free hotline: 1-800-4-CANCER

Government agency that provides free information and operates a hotline from 8 A.M. to midnight, Monday–Friday (EST).

American Cancer Society
1599 Clifton Road, N.E.
Atlanta, Georgia 30329
1-800-952-7664
404-320-3333

A voluntary organization of several thousand local chapters that provides literature on smoking cessation as well as on all aspects of cancer, including prevention, diagnosis, treatment, dealing with psychosocial issues, and so forth. It's advised to contact the unit in your area for specific programs and literature. In addition, they maintain a toll-free information line that draws on an extensive computer database.

Endometriosis/Infertility

Endometriosis Association
8585 North 76th Place
Milwaukee, Wisconsin 53225
414-355-2200

A self-help and support group with over a hundred chapters that provides literature, contact lists, and a bimonthly newsletter. A crisis hotline at the above telephone number may be reached Monday–Friday, 8 A.M. to 5 P.M. (CST).

RESOLVE
1310 Broadway
Somerville, Massachusetts 02144
617-623-0744

This organization offers monthly programs, support groups, counseling, medical referrals, and a newsletter to couples struggling with infertility. Counselors answer calls Monday–Thursday, 9 A.M. to noon and 1 P.M. to 4 P.M. (EST).

The American Society for Reproductive Medicine
1209 Montgomery Highway
Birmingham, Alabama 35216-2809
205-978-5000

This society provides lists and bibliographies of member physicians in your area and printed publications, including booklets about endometriosis and infertility.

General Women's Health

The Boston Women's Health Book Collective
240A Elm Street
Somerville, Massachusetts 02144
617-625-0271

Mailing address:
P.O. Box 192
West Somerville, Massachusetts 02144

A public information center that contains national and international publications concerning health and other issues pertaining to women.

National Women's Health Network
514 Tenth Street, N.W.
Suite 400
Washington, D.C. 20004
202-347-1140

A national organization devoted exclusively to women and health, it publishes a newsletter as well as special news alerts concerning issues requiring immediate attention. Both are available to members.

The Women's International Pharmacy
5708 Monona Drive
Madison, Wisconsin 53716
1-800-279-5708

The Women's International Pharmacy serves physicians and their patients in all states and Canada, compounding prescriptions and providing health care products especially designed for women. The pharmacy also responds to patients' inquiries about premenstrual syndrome, menopausal care, and infertility. It provides a referral network that includes physicians and clinics and welcomes all requests for information. It specializes in compounding natural hormone prescriptions upon physician request.

Heart Disease

American Heart Association
7272 Greenville Avenue
Dallas, Texas 75231
214-373-6300

Provides a variety of materials on heart attacks, strokes, nutrition, exercise, and how to quit smoking. It's best to contact your local affiliate for specific details.

Hysterectomy

**Hysterectomy Educational Resources
and Services Foundation (HERS)**
422 Bryn Mawr Avenue
Bala Cynwyd, Pennsylvania 19004
610-667-7757

This foundation provides free information on alternative treatments for hysterectomy as well as on coping with hysterectomy. It publishes a newsletter, sponsors conferences, and offers telephone counseling. Counseling sessions are conducted by appointment only, Monday–Friday, 9:30 A.M. to noon (EST). Call the 24-hour answering service for an appointment or additional information.

Sexuality

**The American Association of Sex
Educators, Counselors and Therapists
(AASECT)**
435 North Michigan Avenue
Suite 1717
Chicago, Illinois 60611
312-644-0828

Primarily a professional organization providing certification and continuing education programs for its members, it does provide a free listing of member professionals in each state that you may then further evaluate.

**Sex Information and Education Council
of the United States (SIECUS)**
130 West Forty-Second Street
New York, New York 10036
212-819-9770

Serves as an advocacy group and clearinghouse of information that includes an annotated bibliography, publications, lists of organizations providing referrals to qualified sex therapists, and a unique research library and database available to professionals as well as to the general public. Affiliated with New York University.

Osteoporosis

National Osteoporosis Foundation
P.O. Box 96616
Department N-1
Washington, D.C. 20077-7456
1-800-223-9994

Provides information for osteoporosis sufferers.

The BoneMatters Tour
1-800-606-BONE (2663)

This is a motor coach fitted with state-of-the-art bone density testing equipment that is currently traveling across the country to offer osteoporosis screening to various communities. To find out when the bus is scheduled to stop near you, call the toll-free number above.

Urinary Incontinence

Help for Incontinent People (HIP)
P.O. Box 544
Union, South Carolina 29379
1-800-252-3337

The Simon Foundation
P.O. Box 835
Wilmette, Illinois 60091
1-800-23-SIMON

GLOSSARY

ablation Removal or eradication, as by cutting or burning. (For example, endometrial ablation is the removal of the lining of the uterus by laser vaporization.)

adenomyosis Abnormal growth of the lining of the uterus so as to invade the muscular layer; also called internal endometriosis.

adhesion A band of fibrous tissue that sometimes arises abnormally as a result of disease or surgery, thus causing the joining of structures that are not normally bound together.

adnexa A collective term for the ovaries, fallopian tubes, and uterine ligaments.

adrenal gland A small organ located near the kidney and responsible for producing steroids, estrogens, androgens (male sex hormones), progestins, epinephrine and norepinephrine; the latter two are involved in the functioning of the nervous system.

allopathy A philosophy of medicine that focuses on the treatment of disease states by attempting to cure them by producing a condition that is antagonistic to that disease state. Most U.S. medical schools are allopathic schools of medicine. Allopathic physicians have the credential M.D. after their names.

amenorrhea The absence of menses.

analgesic A pain reliever.

androgen Male sex hormone.

anovulatory Lacking the release of an egg or ovum from the ovary.

antioxidant A substance that prevents or delays the harmful effects of oxygen on the cells of the body. Nutrients that function as antioxidants include vitamins C and E and beta-carotene.

arteriosclerosis (atherosclerosis)   A condition in which deposits of cholesterol and other materials form within blood vessels, thus narrowing their diameters; also called "hardening of the arteries."

atrophic vaginitis   A type of vaginal irritation caused by the depletion of estrogen associated with menopause.

atrophy   Wasting away or shrinking in size.

autoimmune   An immune response directed against the body's own tissues.

beta-endorphin   A chemical substance produced by the body that naturally reduces pain and increases a sense of well-being.

bilateral tubal ligation   A sterilization procedure during which the fallopian tubes are clamped, tied, or cut to obstruct the union of sperm and egg.

biopsy   The removal of a sample of tissue for diagnostic examination. (For example, endometrial biopsy is the suctioning out and microscopic evaluation of tissue from the uterine lining.)

calcitonin   A hormone produced by the thyroid gland that is responsible for maintaining calcium balance in the body, specifically by preventing its loss from bone.

carcinoma   Cancer.

castration   The act of rendering a person incapable of reproducing by removing or destroying his or her sex organs; specifically, ovaries in a woman and testes in a man.

CAT scan   Computerized Axial Tomography—a sophisticated type of X ray that uses computer analysis to generate an in-depth view of body tissues.

cautery (cauterize; cauterization)   A procedure used to destroy tissue by cold, heat, or chemicals.

cervix   The lowermost portion of the uterus.

chemotherapy   The use of drugs in the treatment of disease. (For example, drugs used to treat cancer.)

climacteric   Another word for menopause—that era in a woman's life when she may no longer bear children, said to begin once a woman has ceased to menstruate for one year.

clitoris   A small structure located just outside the vagina and capable of erection during sexual arousal; analagous to the penis.

clitoridectomy   The surgical removal of the clitoris.

colposcopy   A procedure using a magnifying lens to examine the cervix and vagina.

condyloma   Also called condyloma acuminata, HPV, or genital warts. A sexually transmitted disease caused by a family of human papilloma viruses that can produce precancerous changes to the cervix. HPV can also infect the external vaginal and anal areas, causing warts in those regions.

cone biopsy   The surgical removal of a cone-shaped area of the cervix for diagnostic and therapeutic purposes.

corpus luteum   The "yellow body" that is created from the follicle in the ovary once its egg has been released; responsible for the secretion of estrogen and progesterone.

cryomyolysis   A method of fibroid destruction using a special probe that penetrates and destroys the tissue by freezing it.

cryosurgery   The destruction of tissue via freezing.

cul-de-sac   The pouch located behind the uterus.

cystocele   A condition that arises when support structures weaken, allowing the bladder to drop down and protrude into the vagina.

D&C   *See* dilation and curettage.

DXA scan   Dual-Energy X-ray Absorbiometry. A method of diagnosing osteoporosis via X ray.

dilation and curettage (D&C)   A surgical procedure during which the cervix is stretched (dilation) to admit instruments that scrape and remove the lining of the uterus (curettage) for diagnostic and therapeutic purposes.

dysfunctional uterine bleeding (DUB)   Abnormal bleeding associated with hormonal imbalance.

dysmenorrhea   Painful menstruation.

dyspareunia   Pain during sexual intercourse.

ectopic pregnancy   The implantation of a fertilized egg outside of the uterus, almost always within the fallopian tube.

endocrine   Pertaining to the system of organs in the body that produce chemical substances called hormones, which then exert their effects on other parts of the body.

endometrial ablation *See* ablation.

endometrioma A large mass containing endometrial tissue.

endovaginal Within the vagina.

endometriosis A condition whereby tissue normally found only in the lining of the uterus is present in other locations throughout the body.

endometrium The tissue comprising the lining of the uterus.

enterocele A hernia or prolapse of intestinal tissue into the vagina.

epithelium The cells that cover the internal and external surfaces of the body.

estrogen The female sex hormone produced by the ovary and the adrenal gland that is responsible for the development of the feminizing characteristics of women as well as playing a role in the menstrual cycle and in pregnancy. Three types are naturally produced by the body: estradiol, estrone, and estriol.

fallopian tubes The structures located between the uterus and ovaries responsible for the transport of the egg; also called oviducts.

fibroid A noncancerous tumor comprised of uterine muscle tissue. There are three types: serosal, intramural, and submucous. Also called a leiomyoma or myoma.

follicle A receptacle within the ovary that houses immature eggs.

follicle stimulating hormone (FSH) Causes the maturation and release of one egg each month from the ovarian follicles.

gonadotrophin releasing factors/hormones (GnRH) Substances having a stimulating effect on the sex hormones.

HPV Human papilloma virus. *See* condyloma.

hemorrhage Bleeding.

homeopathy The philosophy of healing based on the belief that "like cures like." Homeopathic practitioners administer small amounts of substances that produce symptoms similar to those that they are trying to cure.

homeostasis The maintenance of a stable, normal, and balanced body system or internal environment through a system of feedback controls and checks and balances.

hormone A chemical produced at one site in the body that is responsible for the actions of an organ at another site.

human chorionic gonadotrophin (HCG) The hormone responsible for maintaining estrogen and progesterone levels during pregnancy until the placenta takes over.

hyperplasia The growth of normal cells in abnormally large numbers. (For example, endometrial hyperplasia is the overgrowth of the uterine lining under the influences of prolonged estrogen exposure.)

hypertrophy The enlargement of a structure due to an increase in the size of its cells.

hypothalamus A structure in the brain responsible for maintaining body temperature, for mediating sleep and feeding, and for releasing hormones that regulate the menstrual cycle.

hysterectomy The surgical removal of the uterus; variations include subtotal, total, radical, abdominal, laparoscopic, and vaginal.

hysteroscopy A diagnostic test during which a fiberoptic scope is introduced into the body via the cervix to examine the uterus.

iatrogenic illness Physician-induced disease.

in vitro fertilization The union of sperm and egg outside of the body.

incontinence The inability to consciously control urination or defecation. (For example, stress incontinence is the leakage of urine during laughter, coughing, or straining.)

infertility The inability to conceive after one year of unprotected intercourse.

internal endometriosis *See* adenomyosis.

isoflavone A type of phytoestrogen.

LAVH Laparoscopically-Assisted Vaginal Hysterectomy. *See* hysterectomy.

LEEP Loop Electroexcision Procedure. A method of removing diseased cervical tissue without necessitating a hysterectomy or any type of surgical incision.

labia majora/minora The large and small outer and inner lips located at the entrance to the vagina.

laminaria   Rods of sterilized seaweed inserted into the cervix to dilate it, thus facilitating certain procedures, such as vaginal myomectomies.

laparoscopy   A diagnostic test during which a fiberoptic scope is inserted through the navel to view the internal pelvic organs.

laparotomy   The term for open abdominal surgery.

laser   Light amplification by stimulated emission of radiation—a device which transforms light into an intense and highly focused beam capable of generating heat that can cut, coagulate, or vaporize tissue. Types discussed in this book include the "Nd:YAG," "Argon," "KTP," and "CO2" lasers.

leiomyoma   *See* fibroid.

lignan   A type of phytoestrogren.

libido   Sex drive.

luteinizing hormone (LH)   A chemical that facilitates the conversion of a follicle to a corpus luteum.

lymph   A fluid that bathes tissues and is responsible for the transport of certain substances throughout the body.

malignancy   A tendency to progress in severity, often resulting in death, as in cancer.

mammogram   A specialized X ray of the breasts taken to screen for cancer and other pathology.

menarche   The onset of menstruation.

menopause   *See* climacteric.

menstruation   The monthly cycle of hormone production and ovarian activities that prepares the female body for pregnancy, culminating in shedding of the uterine lining and bleeding if conception does not take place.

meridian   An energy channel utilized in Chinese medicine.

metabolism   The sum of all activities that sustain life, including those resulting in the creation of body structures as well as those resulting in tissue destruction with the subsequent release of energy. The rate at which we burn energy is called our metabolic rate.

metastasis   The spread of disease from one organ to another, as in cancer metastasis.

mons pubis   The fleshy mound of tissue covering the pubic bone in women.

morbidity/mortality   Pertaining to disease/death, respectively.

MRI   Magnetic resonance imaging—a high-tech diagnostic test utilizing a powerful magnet and a computer to analyze tissue structures.

multiparity   The condition of having had more than one child.

myolyisis   *See* myoma coagulation.

myoma   *See* fibroid.

myoma coagulation   A process of obliterating a fibroid by piercing it multiple times with a laser or electrical instrument which destroys the tissue and its blood supply.

myomectomy   The surgical excision of uterine fibroids.

myometrium   The muscular, middle layer of the uterus.

neonatal   Pertaining to the newborn.

neoplasia   Pertaining to the abnormal and uncontrollable growth of tissue, as in cancer.

oophorectomy   The surgical removal of the ovary.

os   The opening of the cervix.

osteoblast   A cell that produces bone.

osteoclast   A cell that breaks down bone.

osteoporosis   A condition in which bone weakens and deteriorates as a result of bone destruction exceeding production.

ovary   The organ that produces and houses the female reproductive cells called ova. It is also the site of estrogen and progesterone production.

oviducts   *See* fallopian tubes.

ovulation   The monthly release of an egg from the ovary that will either be followed by pregnancy, if a sperm cell is present to join with it, or menstruation, if conception does not occur.

ovum (pl. ova)   The egg or female reproductive cell.

Pap smear   A screening test for cervical cancer performed by scraping the superficial cells from the cervix during a pelvic examination and subjecting them to laboratory analysis for abnormalities.

parathyroid gland   Four small bodies located in the neck and responsible for maintaining calcium balance.

pelvic inflammatory disease (PID)   An infection, usually sexually transmitted, involving the uterus, ovaries, and/or fallopian tubes.

perineum   The floor of the pelvis. The region located between the pubic bone and the anus.

phytoestrogen   A natural estrogen found in plant material, such as vegetables.

pituitary gland   A pea-sized organ within the brain, responsible for regulating hormones associated with the menstrual cycle. It works in conjunction with the hypothalamus.

placenta   A structure created within the uterus during pregnancy that links the mother's circulation to the developing fetus's, and serves as a source of nutrition and waste elimination.

polyp   A noncancerous, protruding growth. (For example, cervical polyp.)

postpartum   The period immediately after childbirth.

progesterone/progestin   A hormone produced in the ovary, adrenal gland, and placenta (of a pregnant woman) that prepares for and sustains pregnancy.

prolapse   The dropping down of an organ into an abnormal location as a result of a weakening of the support structures that normally hold it in place.

proliferative phase   The stage of the menstrual cycle when the uterine lining is being built up in preparation for pregnancy.

prophylactic   Preventative.

prostaglandin   A chemical carrying out several functions in the body, including the initiation of uterine contractions, which cause menstrual cramps in some women.

qi   A Chinese medicine term for the body's energy.

radiotherapy   The use of potent X rays to destroy abnormal tissue, as in the treatment of cancer.

rectocele   A condition that arises when support structures weaken, allowing the rectum to prolapse into the vagina.

rectovaginal   Pertaining to or communicating with the rectum and the vagina, as in rectovaginal wall.

resectoscope   A surgical device that is inserted into the uterus and used to remove tissue for diagnostic and/or therapeutic purposes.

salpingitis   Infection and inflammation of the fallopian tubes.

salpingo-oophorectomy   The surgical removal of the ovaries and fallopian tubes.

sarcoma   A cancerous tumor; for example, leiomyosarcoma is a cancerous fibroid.

secretory (luteal) phase   The phase of the menstrual cycle following formation of the corpus luteum and progesterone release.

smegma   A cheesy discharge made up of cellular debris and found in the vaginal area.

sonogram   A diagnostic test utilizing sound waves to detect differences in tissue densities and thus to analyze body organs.

speculum   A plastic or metal device inserted during a pelvic exam to separate the walls of the vagina, allowing a clearer view of the cervix.

steroids   A group of substances of similar chemical structure. This family includes the sex hormones.

supracervical   Above the cervix, as in supracervical hysterectomy.

testosterone   The male sex hormone responsible for the development of masculinizing characteristics.

thrombophlebitis   A condition in which a blood clot forms within a vein, leading to its inflammation; results in pain and impaired circulation.

toxic shock syndrome   A potentially fatal bacterial infection usually occurring in menstruating women using tampons; marked by high fever, vomiting, diarrhea, rash, dizziness, sore throat, and other flulike symptoms.

transdermal   Across the skin; as in transdermal estrogen patches—a type of patch that is applied to the skin allowing the systematic release of estrogen into the body through skin penetration.

transformation/transitional zone   An area of the cervix bordering two types of cells and highly susceptible to cervical cancer.

transvaginal   Across the vagina; as in transvaginal ultrasound, whereby the sonographic probe is inserted into the vagina to obtain a better view of certain structures (such as the ovary) than can be obtained otherwise.

tumor   An abnormal growth of tissue that may or may not be cancerous.

ultrasound   *See* sonogram.

urethrocele   A prolapse of the urethra into the vaginal wall.

uterus   The organ of the body within which a fetus develops. It may have other functions that have yet to be clarified by scientists.

xenoestrogen   An estrogenlike substance found in the environment.

BIBLIOGRAPHY

Preface

Budoff, Penny. *No More Menstrual Cramps and Other Good News* (New York: Putnam, 1980), 178–79.

Cutler, Winnifred B. *Hysterectomy: Before and After* (New York: Harper & Row, 1988), 2.

Giustini, F. G., and F. J. Keefer. *Understanding Hysterectomy: A Woman's Guide* (New York: Walker and Company, 1979), 44.

Irwin, Kathleen L., et al. "Hysterectomy among Women of Reproductive Age, United States, Update for 1981–1982," *Morbidity and Mortality Weekly Report: Center for Disease Surveillance Summary for 1986* 35, no. 1 (1986): 1SS–6SS.

Lyons, Albert S., and Joseph R. Petrucelli. *Medicine: An Illustrated History* (New York: Abradale, 1987), 217.

Pokras, Robert, and Vicki G. Hufnagel. "Hysterectomies in the United States: 1965–1984." U.S. Department of Health and Human Services, National Health Survey. *Vital and Health Statistics* 13, no. 92: 1–32.

Ravnikar, Veronica A., and Evelyn Chen. "Hysterectomies: Where Are the Indications?" *Obstetrics and Gynecology Clinics of North America* 21, no. 2 (June 1994): 405–11.

Sandberg, Sonja I., et al. "Elective Hysterectomy: Benefits, Risks, and Costs." *Medical Care* 23, no. 9 (September 1985): 1068.

Scully, Diane. *Men Who Control Women's Health: The Miseducation of Obstetrician-Gynecologists* (Boston: Houghton Mifflin, 1980), 141.

Stokes, Naomi Miller. *The Castrated Woman: What Your Doctor Won't Tell You About Hysterectomy* (New York: Franklin Watts, 1986), 49.

Chapter 1 / The Hysterectomy Controversy

Bachmann, Gloria A. "Hysterectomy: A Critical Review." *Journal of Reproductive Medicine* 35, no. 9 (September 1990): 839–62.

235

Bernstein, Steven, et al. "The Appropriateness of Hysterectomy: A Comparison of Care in Seven Health Plans." *Journal of the American Medical Association* 269, no. 18 (May 12, 1993): 2398–2402.

Bickell, Nina, et al. "Gynecologists' Sex, Clinical Beliefs, and Hysterectomy Rates." *American Journal of Public Health* 84, no. 10 (October 1994): 1649–52.

_____ . "A Matter of Opinion About Hysterectomies: Experts' and Practicing Community Gynecologists' Ratings of Appropriateness." *American Journal of Public Health* 85, no. 8 (August 1995): 1125–28.

Budoff, Penny. *No More Menstrual Cramps and Other Good News* (New York: Putnam, 1980), 178–79.

Bunker, John P. "Elective Hysterectomy: Pro and Con." *New England Journal of Medicine* 295, no. 5 (July 29, 1976): 265.

_____ . "Surgical Manpower: A Comparison of Operations and Surgeons in the United States and in England and Wales." *New England Journal of Medicine* 282, no. 3 (January 15, 1979): 135–44.

Carlson, Karen J., David H. Nichols, and Isaac Schiff. "Indications for Hysterectomy." *New England Journal of Medicine* 328, no. 12 (1993): 856–60.

Carlson, Karen J., Buell A. Miller, and Floyd J. Fowler Jr. "The Maine Women's Health Study: I. Outcomes of Hysterectomy." *Obstetrics and Gynecology* 83 (April 1994): 556–65.

_____ . "The Maine Women's Health Study: II. Outcomes of Nonsurgical Management of Leiomyomas, Abnormal Bleeding, and Chronic Pelvic Pain." *Obstetrics and Gynecology* 83 (April 1994): 566–72.

Cole, Philip, and Joyce Berlin. "Elective Hysterectomy." *American Journal of Obstetrics and Gynecology* 129, no. 2 (September 15, 1977): 117–29.

Subcommittee on Oversight and Investigations of the Committee on Interstate and Foreign Commerce. "Cost and Quality of Health Care: Unnecessary Surgery." (Washington, D.C.: 1976).

Dicker, Richard C., et al. "Hysterectomy Among Women of Reproductive Age: Trends in the United States, 1970–1978." *Journal of the American Medical Association* 248, no. 3 (July 16, 1982): 323–27.

Domenighetti, Gianfranco, and Pierangelo Luraschi. "Hysterectomy and the Sex of the Gynecologist." [Letter]. *New England Journal of Medicine* 313, no. 23 (December 5, 1985): 1482.

Dyck, Frank J., et al. "Effect of Surveillance on the Number of Hysterectomies in the Province of Saskatchewan." *New England Journal of Medicine* 296, no. 23 (June 9, 1977).

Evans, W. A. *Dr. Evans' How to Keep Well Book: A Health Book for the Home* (New York: D. Appleton and Company, 1917), 965–66.

Finkel, Madelon, and David J. Finkel. "The Effect of a Second Opinion Program on Hysterectomy Performance." *Medical Care* 28, no. 9 (September 1990): 776–83.

Geller, S. E., et al. "The Impact of Nonclinical Factors on Practice Variations: The Case of Hysterectomies." *Health Service Review* 30 (February 1996): 729–50.

Grimes, David A. "Shifting Indications for Hysterectomy: Nature, Nurture, or Neither?" [Letter]. *Lancet* 343 (December 17, 1994): 1652–53.

Giustini, F. G., and F. J. Keefer. *Understanding Hysterectomy: A Woman's Guide* (New York: Walker and Company, 1979), 13–14, 39, 47.

Harrison, Michelle. *A Woman in Residence* (New York: Random House, 1982), 32.

Hickey, Martha, and Ian S. Fraser. "Shifting Indications for Hysterectomy." [Letter]. *Lancet* 345 (February 11, 1995): 388–89.

Kjerulff, Kristen H., et al. "Hysterectomy and Race." *Obstetrics and Gynecology* 82, no. 5 (November 1993): 757–64.

Kjerulff, Kristen H., Patricia Langenberg, and Day Guzinski. "The Socioeconomic Correlates of Hysterectomies in the United States." *American Journal of Public Health* 83, no. 1 (January 1993): 106–108.

Lippman, Susan. "Lament for a Lost Uterus." *network* (April 1994): 6–7, 58.

Lyons, Albert S., and R. Joseph Petrucelli. *Medicine: An Illustrated History* (New York: Abradale, 1987), 529.

Notman, Malkah T., and Carol C. Nadelson. *The Woman Patient: Medical and Psychological Interfaces* (New York: Plenum, 1978), 222.

Novak, Edmund R., Georgeanna S. Jones, and Howard Jones. *Novak's Textbook of Gynecology* (Baltimore: Williams & Wilkins, 1975), 113.

Pernick, Martin S. *A Calculus of Suffering: Pain, Professionalism and Anesthesia in Nineteenth-Century America* (New York: Columbia University Press, 1985).

Pokras, Robert, and Vicki G. Hufnagel. "Hysterectomies in the United States: 1965–1984." U.S. Department of Health and Human Services, National Health Survey. *Vital and Health Statistics* 13, no. 92, 3.

Ravnikar, Veronica A., and Evelyn Chen. "Hysterectomies: Where Are the Indications?" *Obstetrics and Gynecology Clinics of North America* 21, no. 2 (June, 1994): 405–11.

Roeske, Nancy C. "Hysterectomy and the Quality of a Woman's Life." [Editorial]. *Archives of Internal Medicine* 139, no. 2 (February 1979): 1467.

Rutkow, Ira M., and George D. Zuidema. "Unnecessary Surgery: An Update." *Surgery* 84, no. 5 (November 1978): 672.

Sandberg, Sonja I. et al. "Elective Hysterectomy: Benefits, Risks, and Costs." *Medical Care* 23, no. 9 (September 1985): 1067.

Scully, Diane. *Men Who Control Women's Health: The Miseducation of Obstetrician-Gynecologists* (Boston: Houghton Mifflin, 1980), 25–60, 103–104, 141–45.

Stage, Sarah. *Female Complaints: Lydia Pinkham and the Business of Women's Medicine* (New York: Norton, 1979), 77–78.

Stokes, Naomi Miller. *The Castrated Woman: What Your Doctor Won't Tell You About Hysterectomy* (New York: Franklin Watts, 1986), 143–50.

Studd, John. "Shifting Indications for Hysterectomy." [Letter]. *Lancet* 345 (February 11, 1995): 388.

Stumpf, Paul G. "Prophylactic Hysterectomy at Oophorectomy in Young Women." [Letter]. *Journal of the American Medical Association* 252, no. 9 (September 7, 1984): 1129.

Wennberg, John, and Alan Gittelsohn. "Variations in Medical Care among Small Areas." *Scientific American* 246, no. 4 (April 1982): 120–34.

Wilcox, Lynne S. et al. "Hysterectomy in the United States: 1988–1990." *Obstetrics and Gynecology* 83, no. 4 (April, 1994): 549–55.

Wright, Ralph C. "Hysterectomy: Past, Present and Future." *Obstetrics and Gynecology* 3, no. 33 (April 1969): 560–63.

Chapter 2 / How Your Reproductive System Really Works

Boston Women's Health Collective, *The New Our Bodies, Our Selves* (New York: Simon & Schuster, 1984), 203–19, 443–47.

Clarke, Edward H., *Sex in Education, or A Fair Chance for Girls* (Boston: Robert Brothers, 1873), 33, as cited in Sarah Stage, *Female Complaints: Lydia Pinkham and the Business of Women's Medicine* (New York: Norton, 1979), 69.

Crouch, James E. *Functional Human Anatomy*. 3d ed. (Philadelphia: Lea and Febiger, 1978), 561–609.

Cutler, Winnefred B. *Hysterectomy: Before and After* (New York: Harper & Row, 1988), 14, 34, 41.

Ezrin, Calvin, John O. Godden, and Robert Volpe. *Systematic Endocrinology*. 2d ed. (New York: Harper & Row, 1979), 258–331.

Guyton, Arthur C., and John E. Hall. *Textbook of Medical Physiology*. 9th ed. (Philadelphia: W. B. Saunders, 1996), 1017–32.

Madaras, Lynda, and Jane Patterson, with Peter Schick. *Womancare: A Gynecological Guide to Your Body* (New York: Avon, 1984), 50–76.

Silverstein, Alvin. *Human Anatomy and Physiology.* 2d ed. (New York: Wiley, 1983), 623–35.

Todd, W. Duane, and Donald F. Tapley, eds. *The Columbia University College of Physicians and Surgeons Complete Guide to Pregnancy* (New York: Crown, 1988), 213.

Chapter 3 / Fibroid Tumors of the Uterus

Andreotti, Rochelle F., et al. "Ultrasound and Magnetic Resonance Imaging of Pelvic Masses." *Surgery, Gynecology and Obstetrics* 166, no. 4 (April 1988): 327–32.

Baird, David, and Christine West. "Medical Management of Fibroids." *British Medical Journal* 296, no. 6638 (June 18, 1988): 1684–85.

Baltarowich, Oksana H., et al. "Pitfalls in the Sonographic Diagnosis of Fibroids." *American Journal of Radiology* 151 (October 1988): 725–28.

Ben-Baruch, G., E. Schiff, Y. Menashe, and J. Menczer. "Immediate and Late Outcome of Vaginal Myomectomy for Prolapsed Pedunculated Submucous Myoma." *Obstetrics and Gynecology* 72, no. 6 (December 1988): 858–60.

Bradham, Douglas, Thomas Stovall, and Chris Thompson. "Use of GnRH Agonist Before Hysterectomy: A Cost Simulation." *Obstetrics and Gynecology* 85, no. 3 (March 1995): 401–6.

Brooks, Philip G., et al. "Resectoscopy: Mastering the Challenges." *Contemporary OB/GYN* (August 1989): 131–48.

Buttram, Veasy, and Robert C. Reiter. "Uterine Leiomyomata: Etiology, Symptomatology and Management." *Fertility and Sterility* 36, no. 4 (October 1981): 433–45.

Carr, Phyllis L., Karen M. Freund, and Sujata Somani. *The Medical Care of Women* (Philadelphia: W. B. Saunders, 1995), 121–25.

Cooke, Cynthia W., and Susan Dworkin. *The* Ms. *Guide to a Woman's Health* (New York: Berkley, 1979), 36–45.

Corfman, Randle S., "Indications for Hysteroscopy." *Obstetrics and Gynecology Clinics of North America* 15, no. 1 (March 1988): 419.

Coutinho, Elsimar, Genevieve Boulanger, Azadian, and Maria Tereza Goncalves. "Regression of Uterine Leiomyomas After Treatment with Gestrinone, An Antiestrogen, Antiprogesterone." *American Journal of Obstetrics and Gynecology* 155, no. 4 (October 1986): 761–67.

Cramer, S. F., et al. "Epidemiology of Uterine Leiomyomas: With an Etiologic Hypothesis." *Journal of Reproductive Medicine* 40 (August 1995): 595–600.

Danforth, David N., and James R. Scott. *Obstetrics/Gynecology* (Philadelphia: Lippincott, 1986), 1079–80.

Droegemueller, William, et al. *Comprehensive Gynecology* (Washington, D.C.: Mosby, 1987), 459–65.

Goldfarb, Herbert A. "Bipolar Laparoscopic Needles for Myoma Coagulation." *Journal of the American Association of Gynecologic Laparoscopists* 2, no. 2 (February 1995): 175–79.

_____ . "D&C Results Improved by Hysteroscopy." *New Jersey Medicine* 86, no. 4 (April 1989): 277–79.

_____ . "Laparoscopic Coagulation of Myoma (Myolysis)." *Infertility and Reproductive Medicine Clinics of North America* 7, no. 1 (January 1996): 129–41.

_____. "Removing Uterine Fibroids Laparoscopically." *Contemporary OB/GYN* 39, no. 2 (February 1994): 50–72.

Goldrath, Milton H. "Vaginal Removal of the Pedunculated Submucous Myoma: The Use of Laminaria." *Obstetrics and Gynecology* 70, no. 10 (October 1987): 670–71.

Goldrath, M., and A. I. Sherman. "Office Hysteroscopy and Suction Curettage: Can We Eliminate the Hospital Diagnostic Dilation and Curettage?" *American Journal of Obstetrics and Gynecology* 152 (1985): 220–29.

Harrison, Michelle. *A Woman in Residence* (New York: Random House, 1982), 35, 59, 216.

Healy, David L., et al. "Toward Removing Uterine Fibroids without Surgery: Subcutaneous Infusion of a Luteinizing Hormone-Releasing Hormone Agonist Commencing in the Luteal Phase." *Journal of Clinical Endocrinology and Metabolism* 63, no. 1 (1986): 619–24.

Hricak, Hedvig. "MRI of the Female Pelvis: A Review." *American Journal of Radiology* 146 (June 1986): 1115–22.

Hricak, Hedvig, et al. "Uterine Leiomyomas: Correlation of MR, Histopathologic Findings, and Symptoms." *Radiology* 158, no. 2 (February 1986): 385–91.

Kistner, Robert. *Gynecology Principles and Practices* (Chicago: Year Book Medical Publishers), 196–209.

Lavy, Gad. "Hysteroscopy as a Diagnostic Aid." *Obstetrics and Gynecology Clinics of North America* 15, no. 1 (March 1988): 61–72.

LiPuma, Joseph P., et al. "Magnetic Resonance Imaging of the Genitourinary Tract." *Urologic Clinics of North America* 13, no. 3 (August 1986): 531–50.

Loffer, Franklin D. "Hysteroscopy with Selective Endometrial Sampling Compared with D&C for Abnormal Uterine Bleeding: The Value of a Negative View." *Obstetrics and Gynecology* 73, no. 1 (January 1989): 169.

_____ . "Laser Ablation of the Endometrium." *Obstetrics and Gynecology Clinics of North America* 15, no. 1 (March 1988): 77–89.

McLachlan, Robert I., David L. Healy, and Henry G. Burger. "Clinical Aspects of LHRH Analogues in Gynaecology: A Review." *British Journal of Obstetrics and Gynaecology* 93, no. 5 (May 1986): 431–54.

Madaras, Lynda, and Jane Patterson, with Peter Schick. *Womancare: A Gynecological Guide to Your Body* (New York: Avon, 1981).

Makarainen, Leo, and Olavi Ylikorkala. "Primary and Myoma-Induced Menorrhagia: Role of Prostaglandins and Effects of Ibuprofen." *British Journal of Obstetrics and Gynaecology* 93, no. 9 (September 1986): 974–78.

Mark, Alexander S., et al. "Adenomyosis and Leiomyoma: Differential Diagnosis with MR Imaging." *Radiology* 163, no. 2 (May 1987): 527–29.

Mendelson, Ellen B., et al. "Gynecologic Imaging: Comparison of Transabdominal and Transvaginal Sonography." *Radiology* 166, no. 2 (February 1988): 321–24.

Napoli, Maryann. "Medical Breakthrough: Laser Hysterectomy." *Ms.* (March 1986), 30–31.

Neuwirth, Robert S. "Hysteroscopic Management of Symptomatic Submucous Fibroids." *Obstetrics and Gynecology* 62, no. 4 (October 1983): 509–11.

Parazzini, Fabio, et al. "Epidemiologic Characteristics of Women with Uterine Fibroids: A Case-Control Study." *Obstetrics and Gynecology* 72, no. 6 (December 1988): 853–57.

Phillips, Douglas R., et al. "Transcervical Electrosurgical Resection of Submucous Leiomyomas for Chronic Menorrhagia." *Journal of the American Association of Gynecologic Laparoscopists* 2, no. 2 (February 1995): 147–53.

Rein, Mitchell, et al. "Progesterone: A Critical Role in the Pathogenesis of Uterine Myomas." *American Journal of Obstetrics and Gynecology* 172 (1995): 14–18.

Ross, Ron K., et al. "Risk Factors for Uterine Fibroids: Reduced Risk Associated with Oral Contraceptives." *British Medical Journal* 293, no. 6543 (August 9, 1986): 359–62.

Russell, Jeffrey B. "History and Development of Hysteroscopy." *Obstetrics and Gynecology Clinics of North America* 15, no. 1 (March 1988): 1–11.

Scheid, T. M. "Endometrial Ablation as an Alternative to Hysterectomy." *Wisconsin Medical Journal* 92 (August 1993): 456–57.

Schmidt, Cecilia. "Applications of GnRH Agnoists for Gyn Patients." *Contemporary OB/GYN* (October 1991): 50–60.

Sener, A. B., et al. "The Effects of Hormone Replacement Therapy on Uterine Fibroids in Postmenopausal Women." *Fertility and Sterility* 65 (February 1996): 354–57.

Shapiro, Bruce S. "Instrumentation in Hysteroscopy." *Obstetrics and Gynecology Clinics of North America* 15, no. 1 (March 1988): 13–21.

Stage, Sarah. *Female Complaints: Lydia Pinkham and the Business of Women's Medicine* (New York: Norton, 1979), 70–71.

Stovall, Thomas, et al. "A Randomized Trial Evaluating Leuprolide Acetate Before Hysterectomy as Treatment for Leiomyomas." *American Journal of Obstetrics and Gynecology* 164, no. 6 (June 1991): 1420–25.

"Uterine Fibroids: Medical Treatment or Surgery?" [Editorial]. *The Lancet* 2, no. 8517 (November 22, 1986): 1197.

"Uterine Leiomyomata." *ACOG Technical Bulletin* 192 (May 1994): 1–9.

Valle, Rafael F. "Future Growth and Development of Hysteroscopy." *Obstetrics and Gynecology Clinics of North America* 15, no. 1 (March 1988): 113–26.

van Leusden, H. A. I. M. "Rapid Reduction of Uterine Myomas After Short-Term Treatment with Microencapsulated D-Trp-LHRH." *Lancet* 2, no. 8517 (November 22, 1986): 1213.

Wamsteker, Kees, Mark Emanuel, and Jan H. de Kruif. "Transcervical Hysteroscopic Resection of Submucous Fibroids for Abnormal Uterine Bleeding: Results Regarding the Degree of Intramural Extension." *Obstetrics and Gynecology* 82, no. 5 (November 1993): 736–40.

Wheeler, James M., and Alan H. DeCherney. "Office Hysteroscopy." *Obstetrics and Gynecology Clinics of North America* 15, no. 1 (March 1988): 29–39.

Willson, J. Robert, and Elsie Reid Carrington. *Obstetrics and Gynecology* (Washington, D.C.: Mosby, 1987), 649–55.

Ylikorkala, O., and Fredrika Pekonen. "Naproxen Reduces Idiopathic But Not Fibromyoma-Induced Menorrhagia." *Obstetrics and Gynecology* 68, no. 1 (July 1986): 10–12.

Chapter 4 / *Endometriosis and Adenomyosis*

Ballweg, Mary Lou, and the Endometriosis Association. *The Endometriosis Sourcebook* (Chicago: Contemporary Books, Inc., 1995).

Barbieri, Robert L. "New Therapy for Endometriosis." *New England Journal of Medicine* 318, no. 8 (February 25, 1988): 512–13.

Bohlman, Mark E., Robert E. Ensor, and Roger C. Sanders. "Sonographic Findings in Adenomyosis of the Uterus." *American Journal of Radiology* 148 (April 1987): 765–66.

Boston Women's Health Collective. *The New Our Bodies, Our Selves* (New York: Simon & Schuster, 1984), 480–81, 500–502.

Breitkopf, Lyle, and Marion Gordon Bakoulis. *Coping with Endometriosis* (New York: Prentice-Hall, 1988).

Carr, Phyllis L., Karen M. Freund, and Sujata Somani. *The Medical Care of Women* (Philadelphia: W. B. Saunders, 1995), 121–25.

Cramer, Daniel W. et al. "The Relation of Endometriosis to Menstrual Characteristics, Smoking, and Exercise." *Journal of the American Medical Association* 255, no. 14 (April 11, 1986): 1904–8.

Davis, Gordon D., and Robert A. Brooks. "Excision of Pelvic Endometriosis with the Carbon Dioxide Laser Laparoscope." *Obstetrics and Gynecology* 72, no. 5 (November 1988): 816–19.

Davis, Gordon D. "Management of Endometriosis and Its Associated Adhesions with the CO_2 Laser Laparoscope." *Obstetrics and Gynecology* 68, no. 3 (September 1986): 422–25.

Droegemueller, William. *Comprehensive Gynecology* (Washington, D.C.: Mosby, 1987), 493–514.

Fayez, Jamil A., Louis M. Collazo, and Cheryl Vernon. "Comparison of Different Modalities of Treatment for Minimal and Mild Endometriosis." *American Journal of Obstetrics and Gynecology* 159, no. 4 (October 1988): 927–31.

Fedele, Luigi, et al. "Serum CA 125 Measurements in the Diagnosis of Endometriosis Recurrence." *Obstetrics and Gynecology* 72, no. 1 (July 1988): 19–22.

Few, Barbara J. "Treating Endometriosis with Nafarelin." *Maternal and Child Nursing* 13, no. 5 (September/October 1988): 323.

Goldfarb, Herbert A. "The Use of the Carbon Dioxide Laser During Laparoscopic Surgery." *New Jersey Medicine* 85, no. 1 (January 1988): pp. 27–28.

Haber, G. M., and Y. F. Behelak. "Preliminary Report on the Use of Tamoxifen in the Treatment of Endometriosis." *American Journal of Obstetrics and Gynecology* 156, no. 3 (March 1987): 582–85.

Henze, Milan R., et al. "Administration of Nasal Nafarelin as Compared with Oral Danazol for Endometriosis." *New England Journal of Medicine* 318, no. 8 (February 25, 1988): 485–89.

Kirshon, Brian, and Alfred Poindexter. "Contraception: A Risk Factor for Endometriosis." *Obstetrics and Gynecology* 71, no. 6 (June 1988): 829–31.

Kistner, Robert W. *Gynecology: Principles and Practices* (Chicago: Year Book Medical Publishers, 1986), 393–414.

"LHRH Analogues in Endometriosis." *Lancet* 2, no. 8514 (November 1, 1986): 1016–18.

Lemay, Andre, et al. "Efficacy of Intranasal or Subcutaneous Luteinizing Hormone-Releasing Hormone Agonist Inhibition of Ovarian Function in the Treatment of Endometriosis." *Obstetrics and Gynecology* 158 (February 1988): 233–36.

Lockhart, W. E., and Karl John Karnaky. "Treatment of Endometriosis." *American Journal of Obstetrics and Gynecology* 154, no. 1 (January 1986): 215–16.

Luciano, Anthony A., R. Nuran Turksoy, and Judith Carleo. "Evaluation of Oral Medroxyprogesterone Acetate in the Treatment of Endometriosis." *Obstetrics and Gynecology* 72, no. 3 (September 1988): 323–26.

McLachlan, Robert I., David L. Healy, and Henry G. Burger. "Clinical Aspects of LHRH Analogues in Gynaecology: A Review." *British Journal of Obstetrics and Gynaecology* 93, no. 5 (May 1986): 431–54.

Mark, Alexander S., et al. "Adenomyosis and Leiomyoma: Differential Diagnosis with MR Imaging." *Radiology* 163, no. 2 (May 1987): 527–29.

Mashahashi, T., et al. "Serum CA 125 Levels in Patients with Endometriosis: Changes in CA 125 Levels During Menstruation." *Obstetrics and Gynecology* 72, no. 3 (September 1988): 328–31.

Nishimura, K., et al. "Endometrial Cysts of the Ovary: MR Imaging." *Radiology* 162, no. 2 (February 1987): 315–18.

Older, Julia. *Endometriosis* (New York: Scribner, 1984).

Peterson, Nancy F., and Joelle Rhoe. "Endometriosis: Obtaining Relief Via 'Near-Contact' Laparoscopy." *AORN Journal* 48, no. 4 (October 1988): 700–707, 710, 712.

Pokras, Robert, and Vicki Hufnagel. "Hysterectomies in the United States: 1965–1984." U.S. Department of Health and Human Services, National Health Survey. *Vital and Health Statistics* 13, no. 92.

Rosenfeld, David L., and Jessica Jacob. "Subsequent Pregnancies in Previously Infertile Women with Endometriosis." *Obstetrics and Gynecology* 72, no. 6 (December 1988): 908–10.

Sampson, J. A. "Intestinal Adenomas of Endometrial Type." *Archives of Surgery* 5 (1922): 217–30.

_____ . "Peritoneal Endometriosis Due to the Menstrual Dissemination of Endometrial Tissue into the Peritoneal Cavity." *American Journal of Obstetrics and Gynecology* 14 (1927): 422.

Steingold, K. A., et al. "Treatment of Endometriosis with a Long-Acting Gonadotropin-Releasing Hormone Agonist," *Obstetrics and Gynecology* 69, no. 3 (March 1987): 403–10.

Togashi, K., et al. "Adenomyosis: Diagnosis with MR Imaging," *Radiology* 166, no. 1 (January 1988): 111–14.

Vasilev, Steven A., et al. "Serum CA 125 Levels in Preoperative Evaluation of Pelvic Masses." *Obstetrics and Gynecology* 71, no. 5 (May 1988): 751–55.

Weinstein, Kate. *Living with Endometriosis: How to Cope with the Physical and Emotional Challenges* (Massachusetts: Addison-Wesley, 1987).

Chapter 5 / Hormonal Imbalance and Dysfunctional Uterine Bleeding

Budoff, Penny. *No More Menstrual Cramps and Other Good News* (New York: Putnam, 1980), 189–93.

Conn, Howard F., et al. *Current Therapy* (Philadelphia: W. B. Saunders, 1981), 904–906.

Ezrin, Calvin, John O. Godden, and Robert Volpe. *Systematic Endocrinology* (Maryland: Harper & Row, 1979), 298–303.

Jeffcoate, Sir Norman. *Jeffcoate's Principles of Gynaecology* (London: Butterworth, 1987), 512–31.

Madaras, Lynda, and Jane Patterson, with Peter Schick. *Womancare: A Gynecological Guide to Your Body* (New York: Avon, 1984), 635–40.

Neeson, Jean, and Connie Stockdale. *The Practitioner's Handbook of Ambulatory Ob/Gyn* (New York: Wiley, 1981), 219–24.

Novak, Edmund R., Georgeanna S. Jones, and Howard Jones. *Novak's Textbook of Gynecology* (Baltimore: Williams & Wilkins, 1981), 777–95.

Worley, Richard J. "Dysfunctional Uterine Bleeding: Clarifying Its Definition, Mechanisms, and Management." *Postgraduate Medicine* 79, no. 3 (February 15, 1986): 101–106.

Zimmerman, Ralf. "Dysfunctional Uterine Bleeding." *Obstetrics and Gynecology Clinics of North America* 15, no. 1 (March 1988): pp. 107–10.

Chapter 6 / The Specter of Cancer

American Cancer Society. "Cancer Facts and Figures—1996."

American Cancer Society. *A Cancer Sourcebook for Nurses* (1981), 79–86.

Barber, Hugh R. K. *Manual of Gynecologic Oncology* (Philadelphia: Lippincott, 1989).

Budoff, Penny. *No More Menstrual Cramps and Other Good News* (New York: Putnam, 1980), 189–93.

Cruickshank, Margaret, and Henry Kitchener. "The Problem with Low-Grade Pap Smears." *Contemporary OB/GYN* (August 1996): 80–93.

Evans, Bergen, ed. *Dictionary of Quotations* (New York: Avenel, 1978), 325.

Fetters, Michael, et al. "Effectiveness of Vaginal Papanicolaou Smear Screening After Total Hysterectomy for Benign Disease." *Journal of the American Medical Association* 275, no. 12 (March 27, 1996): 940–47.

Hankinson, Susan, et al. "Tubal Ligation, Hysterectomy, and Risk of Ovarian Cancer." *Journal of the American Medical Association* 270, no. 23 (December 15, 1993): 2813–18.

Hricak, Hedvig, et al. "Endometrial Carcinoma Staging by MR Imaging." *Radiology* 162, no. 2 (February 1987): 297–305.

"Hysterectomy Prevalence and Death Rates for Cervical Cancer—United States, 1965–1988." *Morbidity and Mortality Weekly Report* 41 (January 17, 1992): 17–20.

Madaras, Lynda, and Jane Patterson, with Peter Schick. *Womancare: A Gynecological Guide to Your Body* (New York: Avon, 1981).

Petrek, Jeanne. *A Woman's Guide to the Prevention, Detection, and Treatment of Cancer* (New York: MacMillan, 1985), 34–92.

Pokras, Robert, and Vicki Hufnagel. "Hysterectomies in the United States: 1965–1984." U.S. Department of Health and Human Services, National Health Survey. *Vital and Health Statistics* 13: 92.

Ross, Ronald K., et al. "Avoidable Nondietary Risk Factors for Cancer." *American Family Physician* 38, no. 2 (August 1988): 153–59.

Sightler, Sterling, et al. "Ovarian Cancer Risk in Women with Prior Hysterectomy: A 14-Year Experience at the University of Miami." *Obstetrics and Gynecology* 78, no. 4 (October 1991): 681–84.

Taylor, Robert, et al. "Atypical Cervical Cytology: Colposcopic Follow-Up Using the Bethesda System." *Journal of Reproductive Medicine* 38, no. 6 (June 1993): 443–47.

Chapter 7 / Uterine Prolapse and Urinary Incontinence

Boston Women's Health Collective. *The New Our Bodies, Our Selves* (New York: Simon & Schuster, 1984).

Jeffcoate, Sir Norman. *Jeffcoate's Principles of Gynaecology* (London: Butterworth, 1987), 260–74.

Madaras, Lynda, and Jane Patterson, with Peter Schick. *Womancare: A Gynecological Guide to Your Body* (New York: Avon, 1984).

Nezhat, Ceana, et al. "Laparoscopic Sacral Colpopexy for Vaginal Vault Prolapse." *Obstetrics and Gynecology* 84, no. 5 (November 1994): 885–88.

Papasakelariou, Cristo, and Benton Baker. "Simplifying Sacrospinous Fixation." *Contemporary OB/GYN* 40, no. 7 (April 1996): 144–49.

Pokras, Robert, and Vicki Hufnagel. "Hysterectomies in the United States: 1965–1984." U.S. Department of Health and Human Services, National Health Survey. *Vital and Health Statistics* 13: 92.

Richardson, David. "Conservative Management of Urinary Incontinence: A Symposium." *Journal of Reproductive Medicine* 38, no. 9 (September 1993) 659–91.

Sharp, Turner. "Sacrospinous Suspension Made Easy." *Obstetrics and Gynecology* 82, no. 5 (November 1993): 873–75.

Speert, Harold. *Iconographia Gyniatrica: A Pictorial Hystory of Gynecology and Obstetrics* (Philadelphia: Davis, 1973), 463–64.

Stage, Sarah. *Female Complaints: Lydia Pinkham and the Business of Women's Medicine* (New York: Norton, 1979).

"Urinary Incontinence." *ACOG Technical Bulletin* 213 (October 1995): 1–11.

Young, Stephen, and Samuel Zylstra. "Managing Vaginal Vault Prolapse with Sacrospinous Fixation." *Contemporary OB/GYN* 40, no. 7 (July 1995): 64–72.

Chapter 8 / When Hysterectomy Is Unavoidable

American College of Obstetricians and Gynecologists. "Estrogen Replacement Therapy." *ACOG Technical Bulletin* 93 (April 1986): 1–5.

_____ . "Prophylactic Oophorectomy." *ACOG Technical Bulletin* 111 (December 1987): 1–5.

Armstrong, Bruce K. "Oestrogen Therapy After the Menopause—Boon or Bane?" *Medical Journal of Australia* 148 (March 7, 1988): 213–14.

Barrett-Conner, Elizabeth. "Postmenopausal Estrogen Replacement and Breast Cancer." *New England Journal of Medicine* 321, no. 5 (August 3, 1989): 319–20.

Brinton, L. A., R. Hoover, and J. F. Fraumeni. "Menopausal Oestrogens and Breast Cancer Risk: An Expanded Case-Control Study." *British Journal of Cancer* 54, no. 5 (November 1986): 825–32.

Bronitsky, Carl, and Susan Stuckey. "Complications of Laparoscopic-Assisted Vaginal Hysterectomy." *Journal of the American Association of Gynecologic Laparoscopists* 2, no. 3 (May 1995): 345–347.

Buring, J. E., et al. "A Prospective Cohort Study of Postmenopausal Hormone Use and Risk of Breast Cancer in U.S. Women." *American Journal of Epidemiology* 125, no. 6 (June 1987): 939–47.

Ernster, Virginia, and Steven Cummings. "Progesterone and Breast Cancer." *Obstetrics and Gynecology* 68, no. 5 (November 1986): 715–17.

Gambrell, R. Don. "Use of Progestogen Therapy." *American Journal of Obstetrics and Gynecology* 156, no. 5 (May 1987): 1304–13.

Gambrell, R. Don, Robert C. Maier, and Barbara I. Sanders. "Decreased Incidence of Breast Cancer in Postmenopausal Estrogen/Progestogen Users." *Obstetrics and Gynecology* 62, no. 4 (October 1983): 435–43.

Harris, Mary, and David Olive. "Changing Hysterectomy Patterns after Introduction of Laparoscopically-Assisted Vaginal Hysterectomy." *American Journal of Obstetrics and Gynecology* 171 (1994): 340–44.

Hidlebaugh, Dennis. "A Health Maintenance Organization's Initial Experience with Laparoscopic-Assisted Vaginal Hysterectomy." *Journal of the American Association of Gynecologic Laparoscopists* 2, no. 3 (May 1995): 311–18.

Hillner, Bruce E., James R. Hollenberg, and Stephen G. Pauker. "Postmenopausal Estrogens in Prevention of Osteoporosis: Benefit Virtually Without Risk if Cardiovascular Effects Are Considered." *American Journal of Medicine* 80, no. 6 (June 1986): 1115.

Horwitz, Ralph I. "Estrogens and Endometrial Cancer: Responses to Arguments and Current Status of an Epidemiologic Controversy." *American Journal of Medicine* 81, no. 3 (September 1986): 503–507.

Hulka, Barbara S. "Replacement Estrogens and Risk of Gynecologic Cancers and Breast Cancer." *Cancer* 60, no. 8 (October 15, 1987): 1960–64.

Judd, Howard. "Efficacy of Transdermal Estradiol." *American Journal of Obstetrics and Gynecology* 156 (May 1987): 1326–31.

Key, T. J. A., and M. C. Pike. "The Dose-Effect Relationship Between 'Unopposed' Oestrogens and Endometrial Mitotic Rate: Its Central Role in Explaining and Predicting Endometrial Cancer Risk." *British Journal of Cancer* 57, no. 2 (February 1988): 205–12.

Lufkin, Edward G., et al. "Estrogen Replacement Therapy: Current Recommendations." *Mayo Clinic Proceedings* 63 (May 1988): 453–60.

Nezhat, Camran, et al. "Hospital Cost Comparison Between Abdominal, Vaginal, and Laparoscopy-Assisted Vaginal Hysterectomies." *Obstetrics and Gynecology* 83, no. 5 (May 1994): 713–16.

Phipps, Jeffrey, et al. "Laparoscopic and Laparoscopically-Assisted Vaginal Hysterectomy: A Series of 114 Cases." *Gynaecological Endoscopy* 2 (1993): 7–12.

Pitkin, Roy. "Operative Laparoscopy: Surgical Advance or Technical Gimmick?" [Editorial]. *Obstetrics and Gynecology* 79, no. 3 (March 1992): 441–42.

Pruitt, Bert, and Robert Stafford. "Advantages of Laparoscopic-Assisted Vaginal Hysterectomy." *Contemporary OB/GYN* (February 1995): 23–30.

Redwine, David. "Laparoscopic Hysterectomy Compared With Abdominal and Vaginal Hysterectomy in a Community Hospital." *Journal of the American Association of Gynecologic Laparoscopists* 2, no. 3 (May 1995): 305–10.

Rohan, Thomas E., and Anthony J. McMichael. "Non-Contraceptive Exogenous Oestrogen Therapy and Breast Cancer." *The Medical Journal of Australia* 148 (March 7, 1988): 217–21.

Shapiro, Samuel, et al. "Risk of Localized and Widespread Endometrial Cancer in Relation to Recent and Discontinued Use of Conjugated Estrogens." *New England Journal of Medicine* 313, no. 16 (October 17, 1985): 969–72.

Utian, Wulf H. "Transdermal Estradiol Overall Safety Profile." *American Journal of Obstetrics and Gynecology* 156, no. 5 (May 1987): 1335–38.

Whitehead, Malcolm I., and David Fraser. "Controversies Concerning the Safety of Estrogen Replacement Therapy." *American Journal of Obstetrics and Gynecology* 156, no. 5 (May 1987): 1313–22.

Wingo, Phyllis A., et al. "The Risk of Breast Cancer in Post-menopausal Women Who Have Used Estrogen Replacement Therapy." *Journal of the American Medical Association* 257, no. 2 (January 9, 1987): 209–15.

Chapter 9 / Coping with the Aftermath

American College of Obstetricians and Gynecologists. "Estrogen Replacement Therapy." *ACOG Technical Bulletin* 93 (April 1986): 15.

American Psychiatric Association. *Diagnostic and Statistical Manual of Mental Disorders*, 3d ed., rev. (Washington, D.C.: 1987), 128–29.

Barrett-Conner, Elizabeth. "Estrogen Replacement and Coronary Heart Disease." *Cardiovascular Clinics* (1989): 159–72.

Barzel, Uriel S. "Estrogens in the Prevention and Treatment of Postmenopausal Osteoporosis." *American Journal of Medicine* 85 (December 1988): 847–49.

Brenner, Paul F. "The Menopausal Syndrome." *Obstetrics and Gynecology* 72, no. 5 (November 1988): 6S–11S.

Budoff, Penny. *No More Hot Flashes and Other Good News* (New York: Putnam, 1983), 114–15.

Castelli, W. "Epidemiology of Coronary Heart Disease: The Framingham Study." *American Journal of Medicine* 76 (1984): 4–12.

Chestnut, Charles, et al. "Alendronate Treatment of Postmenopausal Osteoporotic Women: Effect of Multiple Dosages on Bone Mass and Bone Remodeling." *American Journal of Medicine* 99 (August 1995): 144–52.

"Choice of Drugs for Postmenopausal Osteoporosis." *The Medical Letter* 34, no. 882 (October 30, 1992): 101–2.

"Cholesterol Level in Older Women Reduced by Exercise and HRT." *Clinician Reviews* (May 1996): 66–70.

Colditz, Graham, et al. "Menopause and the Risk of Coronary Heart Disease in Women." *New England Journal of Medicine* 316, no. 18 (April 30, 1987): 1105–10.

"Consensus Development Conference: Prophylaxis and Treatment of Osteoporosis." *British Medical Journal* 295 (October 10, 1987): 914–15.

Criqui, Michael H., et al. "Postmenopausal Estrogen Use and Mortality: Results from a Prospective Study in a Defined, Homogeneous Community." *American Journal of Epidemiology* 128, no. 3 (September 1988): 606–13.

Davis, Lisa, et al. "Tracking Women's Bone Loss," *In Health* 4, no. 3 (May/June 1990): 11.

Dennerstein, Lorraine. "Depression in the Menopause." *Obstetrics and Gynecology Clinics of North America* 4, no. 1 (March 1987): 33–40.

Ditkoff, Edward, et al. "Estrogen Improves Psychological Function in Asymptomatic Postmenopausal Women." *Obstetrics and Gynecology* 78, no. 6 (December 1991): 991–96.

Drinkwater, B. L., et al. "Bone Mineral Content of Amenorrheic and Eumenorrheic Athletes." *New England Journal of Medicine* 311, no. 5 (August 2, 1984): 277–81.

"Eating to Lower Your High Blood Cholesterol." *NIH Publication No. 887-2920*, U.S. Department of Health and Human Services (Washington, D.C.: GPO, September 1987).

Ettinger, Bruce. "Overview of the Efficacy of Hormonal Replacement Therapy." *American Journal of Obstetrics and Gynecology* 156, no. 5 (May 1987): 1298–1301.

Fahraeus, Lars. "The Effects of Estradiol on Blood Lipids and Lipoproteins in Postmenopausal Women." *Obstetrics and Gynecology* 72, no. 5 (November 1988): 18S–22S.

Galsworthy, Theresa, and Patricia Wilson. "Osteoporosis: It Steals More Than Bone." *American Journal of Nursing* 96, no. 6 (June 1996): 27–34.

Gambrell, R. Don. "Estrogen-Progestogen Therapy During Menopause: Renewed Interest in the 1980s." *Postgraduate Medicine* 80, no. 6 (November 1, 1986): 261–67.

Genant, H. K., C. E. Cann, B. Ettinger, and G. S. Gordon. "Quantitative Computerized Tomography of Vertebral Spongiosa: A Sensitive Method for Detecting Early Bone Loss after Oophorectomy." *Annals of Internal Medicine* 97 (1982): 699–705.

Gifford-Jones, W. *What Every Woman Should Know about Hysterectomy* (New York: Funk & Wagnall, 1977), 156–57.

Gould, Dinah. "Hidden Problems after a Hysterectomy." *Nursing Times* (June 4, 1986): 436.

Greenblatt, Robert B. "The Use of Androgens in the Menopause and Other Gynecologic Disorders." *Obstetrics and Gynecology Clinics of North America* 14, no. 1 (March 1987): 251–67.

Helstrom, L., et al. "Sexuality After Hysterectomy: A Factor Analysis of Women's Sexual Lives Before and After Subtotal Hysterectomy." *Obstetrics and Gynecology* 81, no. 3 (March 1993): 357–62.

Hillner, Bruce, James P. Hollenberg, and Stephen G. Pauker. "Postmenopausal Estrogens in the Prevention of Osteoporosis: Benefit Virtually Without Risk if Cardiovascular Effects Are Considered." *American Journal of Medicine* 80, no. 6 (June 1986): 1115.

Hreshchyshyn, Myroslaw, et al. "Effects of Natural Menopause, Hysterectomy, and Oophorectomy on Lumbar Spine and Femoral Neck Bone Densities." *Obstetrics and Gynecology* 72, no. 4 (October 1988): 631–37.

Jensen, Jytte, and Claus Christiansen. "Effects of Smoking on Serum Lipoproteins and Bone Mineral Content During Postmenopausal Hormone Replacement Therapy." *American Journal of Obstetrics and Gynecology* 159, no. 4 (October 1988): 820–25.

Judd, Howard, and Wulf Utian. "Current Perspectives in the Management of the Menopausal and Postmenopausal Patient." *American Journal of Obstetrics and Gynecology* 156, no. 5 (May 1987): 1279–1356.

Judd, Howard. "Efficacy of Transdermal Estradiol," *Obstetrics and Gynecology* 156 (May 1987): 1326–31.

Kessenich, Cathy. "Early Detection, Prevention Are Best Defense: Osteoporosis Cycle." *Advance for Nurse Practitioners* (August 1996): 17–20.

_____ . "Update on Pharmacologic Therapies for Osteoporosis." *Nurse Practitioner* 21, no. 8 (August 1996): 19–24.

Kiel, Douglas P., et al. "Hip Fracture and the Use of Estrogens in Postmenopausal Women: The Framingham Study." *New England Journal of Medicine* 317, no. 19 (November 5, 1987): 1169–74.

Knopp, Robert H. "The Effects of Postmenopausal Estrogen Therapy on the Incidence of Arteriosclerotic Vascular Disease." *Obstetrics and Gynecology* 72, no. 5 (November 1988): 23S–30S.

Lalinec-Michaud, Martine, and Frank Engelsmann. "Anxiety, Fears and Depression Related to Hysterectomy." *Canadian Journal of Psychiatry* 30 (February 1985): 44–47.

_____ . "Depression and Hysterectomy: A Prospective Study." *Psychosomatics* 25, no. 7 (July 1984): 550–58.

Lalinec-Michaud, Martine, et al. "Depression After Hysterectomy." *Psychosomatics* 29, no. 3 (Summer 1988): 307–13.

Lievertz, Randolph W. "Pharmacokinetics of Estrogens." *American Journal of Obstetrics and Gynecology* 156, no. 5 (May 1987): 1289–93.

Liberman, Uri, et al. "Effect of Oral Alendronate on Bone Mineral Density and the Incidence of Fractures in Postmenopausal Osteoporosis." *New England Journal of Medicine* 333, no. 22 (November 30, 1995): 1437–43.

Lindemann, E. "Observations on Psychiatric Sequelae to Surgical Operations on Women." *American Journal of Psychiatry* 98 (1941): 132–37.

Lindsay, Robert. "Estrogen Therapy in the Prevention and Management of Osteoporosis." *American Journal of Obstetrics and Gynecology* 156, no. 5 (May 1987): 1347–51.

_____ . "Managing Osteoporosis: Current Trends, Future Possibilities." *Geriatrics* 42, no. 3 (March 1987): 35–40.

Lufkin, Edward, et al. "Estrogen Replacement Therapy: Current Recommendations," *Mayo Clinic Proceedings* 63 (May 1988): 453–60.

Luoto, Riitta, et al. "Cardiovascular Morbidity in Relation to Ovarian Function After Hysterectomy." *Obstetrics and Gynecology* 85, no. 4 (April 1995): 515–22.

Mack, T. M., et al. "Estrogens and Endometrial Cancer in a Retirement Community." *New England Journal of Medicine* 294, no. 23 (June 3, 1976): 1262–67.

Marcus, R., et al. "Menstrual Function and Bone Mass in Elite Women Distance Runners." *Annals of Internal Medicine* 102, no. 2 (February 1985): 158–63.

Mastrangelo, Rosemary. "The Silent Disease: Diagnosing and Treating Osteoporosis." *Advance for Nurse Practitioners* (April 1994): 23–24.

Moquette-Magee, Elaine. *Eat Well for a Healthy Menopause* (New York: John Wiley & Sons, 1996).

Morgan, Susanne. *Coping With a Hysterectomy: Your Own Choice, Your Own Solutions* (New York: Dial, 1982), 148.

Nachtigall, Lila E. "Cardiovascular Disease and Hypertension in Older Women." *Obstetrics and Gynecology Clinics of North America* 14, no. 1 (March 1987): 89–103.

"New Treatment Option for Osteoporosis." *American Journal of Nursing* 96, no. 2 (February 1996): 53–54.

Notelovitz, Morris. "Climacteric Medicine: Cornerstone for Midlife Health and Wellness." *Public Health Reports Supplement* (July/August 1986): 116–23.

_____ . "Exercise, Nutrition, and the Coagulation Effects of Estrogen Replacement on Cardiovascular Health." *Obstetrics and Gynecology Clinics of North America* 14, no. 1 (March 1987): 121–39.

Oldenhave, A., et al. "Hysterectomized Women with Ovarian Conservation Report More Severe Climacteric Complaints Than Do Normal Women of Similar Age." *American Journal of Obstetrics and Gynecology* 168 (March 1993): 765–71.

Pak, Charles, et al. "Treatment of Postmenopausal Osteoporosis with Slow-Release Sodium Fluoride: Final Report of a Randomized Controlled Trial." *Annals of Internal Medicine* 123, no. 6 (September 15, 1995): 401–408.

Pogrund, Hyman, Ronald A. Bloom, and Jacob Menczel. "Preventing Osteoporosis: Current Practices and Problems." *Geriatrics* 41, no. 5 (May 1986): 55–71.

Polan, Mary Lake. "Value of Early Screening for Osteoporosis." *Contemporary OB/GYN* 39 (June 15, 1994): 63–67.

"Postmenopausal Hormone Therapy: Weighing the Risks and Benefits." *HealthFacts—Center for Medical Consumers* 16, no. 144 (May 1991): 1–6.

Rebar, Robert, and Ilene Spitzer. "The Physiology and Measurement of Hot Flushes." *American Journal of Obstetrics and Gynecology* 156, no. 5 (May 1987): 1284–87.

Reeve, J., et al. "Anabolic Effect of Human Parathyroid Hormone Fragment on Trabecular Bone Involutional Osteoporosis: A Multicenter Trial." *British Medical Journal* 280, no. 6228 (June 7, 1984): 1340–44.

Richards, D. H. "A Post-Hysterectomy Syndrome." *Lancet* 2, no. 7887 (October 26, 1974): 983–85.

Riggs, B. Lawrence. "Pathogenesis of Osteoporosis." *American Journal of Obstetrics and Gynecology* 156, no. 5 (May 1987): 1342–46.

Rivlin, Richard S. "Osteoporosis: Nutrition." *Public Health Reports Supplement* (July/August 1986): 131–36.

Sarrel, Philip M. "Estrogen Replacement Therapy." *Obstetrics and Gynecology* 72, no. 5 (November 1988): 2S–5S.

_____ . "Sexuality in the Middle Years." *Obstetrics and Gynecology Clinics of North America* 14, no. 1 (March 1987): 49–61.

Schmidt, Peter, and David Rubinow. "Mood and the Perimenopause." *Contemporary OB/GYN* 39 (June 15, 1994): 68–75.

Sobel, Solomon. "Osteoporosis: Regulatory View." *Public Health Reports Supplement* (July/August 1986): 1369.

Stampfer, Meir J., et al. "A Prospective Study of Postmenopausal Estrogen Therapy and Coronary Heart Disease." *New England Journal of Medicine* 313, no. 17 (October 24, 1985): 1044–48.

Steinberg, Karen K. "Women's Health: Osteoporosis—Introductory Remarks." *Public Health Reports Supplement* (July/August 1986): 1257.

Teran, Ana-Zully, Robert B. Greenblatt, and Jaswant S. Chaddha. "Changes in Lipoproteins with Various Sex Steroids." *Obstetrics and Gynecology Clinics of North America* 14, no. 1 (March 1987): 107–17.

Tufts University School of Medicine and CME Partnership. *Practitioner Update on Diagnosis and Treatment of Osteoporosis* (New York: SCP Communications, 1995).

Utian, Wulf H. "The Fate of the Untreated Menopause." *Obstetrics and Gynecology Clinics of North America* 14, no. 1 (March 1987): 1–11.

———. "Transdermal Estradiol Overall Safety Profile." *American Journal of Obstetrics and Gynecology* 156 (1987): 1335–38.

Watts, Nelson B. "Osteoporosis." *American Family Physician* 38, no. 5 (November 1988): 193–205.

Webb, Christine, and Jenifer Wilson-Barnett. "Hysterectomy: Dispelling the Myths— Parts I and II." *Nursing Times* (November 23/30, 1983): 446, 524.

Wigfall-Williams, Wanda. *Hysterectomy: Learning the Facts, Coping with the Feelings, Facing the Future* (New York: Kesend, 1986), 49.

Wilson, Peter W. F., Robert J. Garrison, and William P. Castelli. "Postmenopausal Estrogen Use, Cigarette Smoking, and Cardiovascular Morbidity in Women Over 50: The Framingham Study." *New England Journal of Medicine* 313, no. 17 (October 24, 1985): 1038–43.

Youngs, David D., and Anke A. Ehrhardt. *Psychosomatic Obstetrics and Gynecology* (New York: Appleton-Century-Crofts, 1980), 255–64.

Ziel, H. K., and W. D. Finkle. "Increased Risk of Endometrial Carcinoma among Users of Conjugated Estrogens." *New England Journal of Medicine* 293, no. 23 (December 4, 1975): 1167–70.

Chapter 10 / Alternative and Adjunct Therapies and the Role of Nutrition

Burton Goldberg Group. *Alternative Medicine—The Definitive Guide* (Washington: Future Medicine Publishing, 1994).

Eisenberg, D. M., et al. "Unconventional Medicine in the United States: Prevalence, Costs, and Patterns of Use." *New England Journal of Medicine* 328 (1993): 246–52.

French, Melody. "The Power of Plants." *Advance for Nurse Practitioners* (July 1996): 16–21.

Golden, B. R., et al. "Estrogen Excretion Patterns and Plasma Levels in Vegetarian and Omnivorous Women." *New England Journal of Medicine* 307 (1982): 1542–47.

———. "Effect of Diet on Excretion of Estrogens in Pre- and Post-Menopausal Women." *Cancer Research* 41 (1981): 3771–73.

Greif, Judith, and Beth Ann Golden. *AIDS Care at Home: A Guide for Caregivers, Loved Ones, and People with AIDS.* (New York: John Wiley & Sons, 1994), 295–304.

Hill, M. J. "Gut Bacteria and Aetiology of Cancer of the Breast." *Lancet* 2 (1971): 472–73.

Hoffman, Ronald. *Tired All The Time* (New York: Pocket Books, 1993), 59–69.

Lichtman, R. "Perimenopausal and Postmenopausal Hormone Replacement Therapy. Part 2. Hormonal Regimens and Complementary and Alternative Therapies." *Journal of Nurse Midwifery* 41 (May/June 1996): 195–210.

Moquette-Magee, Elaine. *Eat Well for a Healthy Menopause* (New York: John Wiley & Sons, Inc., 1996).

Vliet, Elizabeth Lee. *Screaming to be Heard—Hormonal Connections Women Suspect and Doctors Ignore* (New York: M. Evans and Company, 1995).

Yudkin, J., and O. Eisa. "Dietary Sucrose and Oestradiol Concentration in Young Men." *Annals of Nutrition and Metabolism* 32 (1988): 53–55.

Epilogue

Evans, Bergen, ed. *Dictionary of Quotations* (New York: Avelen, 1978), 94.

Llewellyn-Jones, Derek. *Everywoman: A Gynaecological Guide for Life* (London: Faber and Faber, 1971).

Scully, Diane. *Men Who Control Women's Health: The Miseducation of Obstetrician-Gynecologists* (Boston: Houghton Mifflin, 1980).

SOURCES

FIGURES

2.1   Syntex Laboratories, Inc., Palo Alto, CA., Copyright 1985.

3.1   Kistner, Robert, *Gynecology: Principles and Practice, 4th ed.* (Chicago: Year Book Medical Publishers, 1986), p. 197.

3.2   Richard Wolf Medical Instruments Corporation, Rosemont, Illinois.

3.3   Kistner, Robert, *Gynecology: Principles and Practices, 4th ed* (Chicago: Year Book Medical Publishers, 1986), p. 203.

3.4   Richard Wolf Medical Instruments Corporation, Rosemont, Illinois.

4.1   Copyright 1988. Reprinted with permission of the American Society for Reproductive Medicine.

4.2   Copyright 1988. Reprinted with permission of the American Society for Reproductive Medicine.

4.3   Copyright 1988. Reprinted with permission of the American Society for Reproductive Medicine.

4.4   From: The American Society for Reproductive Medicine: Revised American Society for Reproductive Medicine Classification of Endometriosis: 1988. Fertil. Steril. 43:351, 1985. Reproduced with permission of the publisher, The American Society for Reproductive Medicine.

8.1   Sarrel, Philip, "Estrogen Replacement Therapy," *Obstetrics and Gynecology* (1988), 72:5, p. 3S.

8.3   Sarrel, Philip, "Estrogen Replacement Therapy," *Obstetrics and Gynecology* (1988), 72:5, p. 3S.

Figures 2.2, 2.3, 2.4, 7.1, 8.1 and 8.2 are original drawings by Brian Pendley.

TABLES

4.1   Droegmueller, William, *Comprehensive Gynecology,* (Washington, DC.: Mosby, 1987), p. 501.

6.1   American Cancer Society, "Cancer Facts & Figures—1996"

9.2   From *Eat Well for a Healthy Menopause* by Elaine Moquette-Magee, copyright 1996 by Elaine Moquette-Magee. Reprinted by permission of John Wiley and Sons, Inc.

10.1   From *Eat Well for a Healthy Menopause* by Elaine Moquette-Magee, copyright 1996 by Elaine Moquette-Magee. Reprinted by permission of John Wiley and Sons, Inc.

10.2   From *Eat Well for a Healthy Menopause* by Elaine Moquette-Magee, copyright 1996 by Elaine Moquette-Magee. Reprinted by permission of John Wiley and Sons, Inc.

INDEX

ABOUT THE AUTHORS

Dr. Herbert Goldfarb received his M.D. from New York University School of Medicine and served a residency at NYU Bellvue Medical Center in Obstetrics and Gynecology. He then joined the faculty of New York University School of Medicine, but took time out to serve in the United States Military during the Vietnam conflict. He returned to practice in Montclair, New Jersey, where he founded the Montclair Reproductive Center.

In 1985, Dr. Goldfarb was the first physician to perform operative laser laporoscopy in the New York metropolitan area and was the first in New Jersey to do operative hysteroscopy for uterine bleeding ablation. Dr. Goldfarb is a leader in the field of minimally invasive surgery and has lectured throughout the Continental United States, Europe, and Asia.

In 1990, he introduced the procedure of myoma coagulation to destroy fibroids through minimally invasive surgical techniques described in this book.

Dr. Goldfarb is in active private practice and is committed to helping women avoid unwanted hysterectomies, whenever possible and practical.

He can be reached through the Internet at www.hgoldfarb.com

Judith Greif, R.N., F.N.P., C., M.S., is a family nurse practitioner at Rutgers University in New Brunswick, New Jersey. She is on the faculties of Seton Hall University, Pace University, and Columbia University Graduate Schools of Nursing as a Clinical Professor and Instructor in Clinical Nursing. She is the co-author of *AIDS Care at Home: A Guide for Caregivers, Loved Ones, and People with AIDS* and with Dr. Goldfarb is the co-author of *Overcoming Infertility: Twelve Couples Share Their Success Stories.* She currently resides in East Brunswick, New Jersey, with her husband, Joe, and their daughter, Samantha.